YOGA FOR REJUVENATION

Shows how to restore youthful vigour and suppleness using the interpretation and practice of the universal philosophy of yoga.

YOGA
FOR REJUVENATION
Revitalizing Techniques of the Yogis

by

Nergis Dalal

Illustrated by Ian Jones

THORSONS PUBLISHERS LIMITED
Wellingborough, Northamptonshire

First published February 1984
Second Impression May 1984

British Library Cataloguing in Publication Data

Dalal, Nergis
    Yoga for rejuvenation.
    1. Yoga
    I. Title
    181'.45   B132.Y6

    ISBN 0–7225–0771–2

Printed and bound in Great Britain

ACKNOWLEDGEMENTS

My grateful thanks to Dr Swami Gitananda of Ananda Ashram, Pondicherry, for his constant encouragement and for permission to use material from his courses.

CONTENTS

INTRODUCTION

Yoga, they say, is like the spokes of a wheel, and people come to it in many ways and for many different reasons. Mine was pain. For many, many years I suffered such severe back pain that I was virtually crippled. Visits to doctors yielded no results. I was put into traction, spent weeks lying flat on a hard bed, and went through various forms of heat treatment — all to no avail. The pain continued. The doctors told me, 'You can have an operation, and we cannot guarantee success, or you can learn to live with the pain.' I lived with the pain by consuming ever-increasing doses of pain killers which somehow carried me through each day. That was when I picked up a small book on yoga at the airport. Many of the asanas seemed similar to the exercises I had been told to do by the chiropractor. When I tried some of them I was astonished to find that my spine seemed absolutely inflexible: rigid, unbending and painful. How could I ever bend, twist and flex my body into these extraordinary poses? I began slowly to attempt some of the easier ones and to my delight discovered that even a modified version of an asana gave considerable relief to back pain and tension.

Twenty years and several instructors later, my spine is supple, flexible and fully articulated. I have no more pain. I live a full and active life. In gratitude, I decided to teach others what I had learnt. Yoga is for everyone who wants to live a better, healthier, more integrated life. Negative attitudes become positive, and the mind becomes calm and centred in tranquillity. Youthfulness is restored and the body is kept clean, strong and healthy. All that is needed to achieve this is patience, perseverance and courage. In yoga can be found the way to conquer disease, debility, poor health and old age. Let this timeless wisdom of the ancient Rishis bring harmony and health to all mankind.

1

WHAT IS YOGA?

Although yoga is so popular in the West today, there are still many misconceptions about it. When I was writing a series of articles for a health magazine about yoga, a reader wrote in to say she was disappointed with the monthly articles on yoga. 'If your magazine is going to have a religious slant,' she wrote, 'let's hear about peace that other religions offer. If your magazine continues to preach yoga I feel I will have to cancel my subscription and I would encourage all my Christian friends not to subscribe.'

In reply, the editor quoted from *Yoga in Ten Lessons* written by a Benedictine monk, Brother J.M. Dechanet:

> The Yogi seeks perfection in the balanced interplay in him of these three powers, an activity on which the harmony of his being, the development of his personality and the elevation of his inner life depend. He likes to think of divine grace as informing his energies and transposing their activity on a higher, supernatural and divine plane. He does everything he can to dispose his faculties, body, soul and spirit, so that a power coming from on high can take possession.

Yoga in short, is not a religion but a great philosophy, an art, a science, and a way of life, aimed at developing a perfect balance between the body and the mind and between the individual self and the cosmos. It came into being several thousand years ago, invented by great sages who aimed at complete mastery of the body so that the mind could be freed for meditation and other higher spiritual practices. They believed that a body which was ill, infirm, weak or diseased, affected the mind which found itself fettered and earth-bound. When the body was made healthy, supple and free from illness and disease, then the mind too became illuminated, ready to pursue its goal of union with the divine or the *atman* which it is believed is here, within each human being. The Yogi then achieved his final goal: the realization of the Self which was one with all creation.

In the *Shvetaashvatara Upanishad* it is said that disease and old age do not come to the Yogi whose body is supple and healthy and whose mind has been made pure by the practice of yoga.

In the early years the knowledge of yoga was confined to monasteries and ashrams but gradually it spread, taught by gurus who were themselves realized beings. Among the most important sources of literature on yoga is the much quoted and translated *Yoga Sutras of Patanjali*.

The word yoga means 'union' from the Sanskrit word 'yug' meaning to join. Although there are many different types of yoga such as Jnana Yoga (the yoga of knowledge), Karma Yoga (the yoga of service), Bhakti Yoga (the yoga of devotion), Mantra Yoga (the yoga of recitation of sacred words) and so on, this book is concerned with *Hatha Yoga* — the yoga of physical health which combines *asanas* (firm postures), *pranayama* (the control of breath), *kriyas* (movements repeated rhythmically) and *mudras* (neuro-muscular stimulators to pressure glandular secretions) combined with certain relaxation techniques in order to produce total health of body and mind. Hatha Yoga is the base from which the transition is made into Raja Yoga, the Royal path to spiritual illumination, in which both the body and the mind are used to attain a state of pure knowledge and beatitude. Raja Yoga cannot be attained without much practice for many hours a day.

Hatha Yoga, however, is within the grasp of all those who earnestly seek to make the body healthy, full of vital energy, youthful and free from illness and disease. The mind too becomes poised, balanced and in control, able to withstand the stresses and strains of modern life. Scientific research has proved that constant worry, stress and anxiety can produce a variety of illnesses such as diarrhoea, constipation, high blood pressure, colitis, ulcers, asthma, heart attacks and even cancer. When yoga is practised properly it becomes a way to restore balance, mental and physical health, a strong nervous system and an endocrine system that functions perfectly, ensuring health, longevity, supreme intelligence and efficiency. Hatha Yoga teaches us how to utilize the flow of life force to the maximum.

According to Sanskrit texts the word Hatha is divided into two syllables: *Ha* meaning sun or positive energy and *Tha* meaning moon or negative energy. When the two forces join and work together in harmony, the two currents cause complete equilibrium and balance of body and mind.

'Mastery of the body and the breath are an undoubted aid to those concerned with their spiritual evolution. For by having full control over the physical condition the body becomes calm, allowing the mind to be directed inwardly more easily in perfect tranquillity to achieve a higher spiritual level.' Hatha Yoga then is the first step towards achieving spiritual evolution.

What does it mean to grow old?
There are Yogis in India who seem ageless — vigorous, healthy, full of vitality and capable of doing a full day's work. My own guru, Dr Swami Gitananda, who is 75, has just completed a long trek into the high Himalayas. He works a fifteen-hour day, has thick glossy hair, bright eyes, a smooth rosy skin and positively bounces with energy. He is a total vegetarian, does not smoke, drink alcohol or take drugs in any form. 'Time's defacing fingers' seem to have passed him by.

On the other hand, I have seen young men and women, still in their early twenties with slumped shoulders, drooping necks, caved-in chests and pale, wrinkled faces. They stagger around as if they have not even sufficient energy to drag their feet along. They seem to gasp for air and appear to be in the last stages of mental and physical infirmity.

Growing old is inevitable but yoga prevents all the symptoms of ageing that make old age so miserable. 'Growing old youthfully' becomes possible. When the body begins to slow down and deteriorate, the heart doesn't pump blood so efficiently, arteries narrow and stiffen and there is greater resistance to blood flow in the organs. The delivery of nutrients to the cells becomes defective and all physiological processes become sluggish, resulting in various inflammatory processes, hypertension and the loss of sexual powers. Women acquire dowager's humps and fat accumulates on hips, thighs, neck, buttocks and stomach. There is wrinkling of the skin, loss of hair and a lack of suppleness and mobility. An actor imitating an old man will walk stiffly, stooping a little and perhaps limping, head and hands shaking with infirmity. The spring has gone, the elasticity of youth is no more. Worse still, with old age can come incontinence — the inability to control urine and faeces — and the old person becomes a burden, a sick, senile and incompetent parent or spouse.

All these changes, however, need not and should not, occur. Linear age is inevitable but we can grow old still in full possession of all our faculties, both mental and physical, and still healthy, active, and with no decline in mental faculties, only a slight and inevitable reduction in physical strength. This should be the ideal and this is possible with a regular and systematic practice of yoga.

Yoga and other systems of physical culture

While yoga produces a supple, healthy body and a mind that is calm and poised, it does not develop muscles as do other sports and exercises. These muscles however, often develop in a one-sided manner and athlete's heart is well-known. In many ashrams in India there are young men and women from the West — ballet dancers, sportsmen and athletes, karate and judo experts — and all of them have damaged backs or knees, torn ligaments, bones that have broken and been re-set and muscles that have been dangerously over-extended. An active open-air life is good, accompanied by deep breathing, but competition and concentration on speed can build up toxins inside the body and damage nerves, muscles and bones. There is increased tension, the heart palpitates, the pulse races, breathing is fast and perspiration increases. If this continues for any length of time, then resistance and powers of recuperation diminish. Many once-famous sportsmen, for example wrestlers and boxers, are physical wrecks by the time they retire. Ordinary sports and physical exercises affect only external muscles but the inner organs need exercise as well. Although deep breathing is necessary in most sports it is often spasmodic and jerky instead of smooth and rhythmic. Energy is expended in sport but accumulated in Hatha Yoga, in a gigantic storehouse to be drawn upon as necessary. After every yoga session one should get up rested, relaxed and full of energy — all set up, in fact, to face the day. 'I am a better violinist,' said Yehudi Menhuin, 'because of yoga.'

All this does not mean that those who practise yoga must give up sport and other forms of physical exercise. Walking and swimming are both excellent exercises and complement the yoga routine. Any other form of physical exercise should be practised after an interval of two hours or more and not at the same time as yoga.

How yoga affects internal processes

The health of the human body depends mainly on the healthy condition of internal glands and tissues, the thorough elimination of waste matter from the body and the elastic condition of muscles. Many asanas give the internal organs a unique massage, forcing them to perform better. The alternate stretching and contracting movements of the asanas help muscles to retain their tone and keep bones strong and lung tissue healthy. The heart is strengthened and made more resistant by being subjected to alternate pressures, thus improving the circulation of blood to the body. In the upside-down postures blood flows to the heart without the straining against gravity, and sluggishness of the bowels and constipation are cured. The stomach muscles fall into their proper position, helping to flatten and strengthen a protruding belly, and the thyroid gland is activated. Deep controlled breathing increases the oxygen turnover in the body. Four doctors of the VA Hospital at Buffalo, New York and the School of Medicine of the State University of New York at Buffalo confirmed what had already been proved, that oxygen deprivation contributes to symptoms like those of senility — poor memory, lessened ability to do abstract thinking and mental sluggishness. In fact more than a generation ago, Dr Ross A. McFarland of Harvard University, found there were striking similarities in mental handicaps of the senile and oxygen-deprivation. Yoga pranayama keeps enough oxygen in the brain to preserve mental alertness and promote emotional stability.

Inadequate functioning of any of the endocrine glands can cause the most serious disorders but specific yoga asanas benefit the pituitary and pineal glands, the thyroid, the thymus and the sex glands. The network of nerves branching out from the spinal cord to all parts of the body are strengthened and activated while the spine is kept strong and elastic. Forward, backward and numerous forms of torso-twisting positions are used to relieve tension along the spine and to bring a massive supply of blood to the appropriate spinal area. The spine requires good circulation for the manufacture of red and white blood cells in the marrow of the bones and for the supply of blood to the spinal nerves and cord. Poor circulation is bad for the spine and for the body as a whole.

The complete elimination of waste matter in the body is promoted by yoga asanas which not only massage and activate internal muscles for peristaltic activity but also keep internal organs in their proper places in the abdominal cavity, preventing prolapse of the stomach, intestines, vagina and kidneys.

As weapons against premature old age, the asanas, pranayamas and relaxation techniques are invaluable, stimulating mental vigour, nourishing skin and facial tissues and recharging a tired body, just as a battery recharges an engine.

The importance of pranayama

Without pranayama — the science of the control of the breath — there can be no yoga. Every asana has its own breath pattern and breathing forms the basis for all yoga practice. Most people have no idea how to breathe. To breathe properly is to revitalize every nerve, organ and muscle in the body. Life is breath and the cessation of breath is death. Every activity of the body, from digestion and movement to the power of creative thinking, depends on a good supply of oxygen to the brain and tissues. Shallow, quick breathing will produce sickness and ill health. When lungs are filled with stale air the body is starving for oxygen. Pranayama restores order and equilibrium in the positive and negative currents of the body. Most people breathe about 15 times a minute and a shallow breath takes in around 20 cubic inches (328 cubic centimetres) of air. A deep yogic breath can take in 100 cubic inches (1639 cubic centimetres) of air while the breath is slowed down to once or twice a minute, thus calming the whole system and bringing about tranquillity. We breathe rapidly when we are excited, frightened or upset. Slowing the breath automatically calms down the nervous system. Breath control can increase the circulation of blood, revitalize starving tissues and rejuvenate the whole body.

How to begin a practice of yoga

Although yoga needs no equipment nor special apparatus there are certain necessary conditions for a good practice.

1. Clean the body by having a warm shower before your practice. Do not have a hot bath before starting any yoga. Wear clean, loose clothes without anything tight around waist, chest or neck. In fact the fewer clothes you wear the better.

2. The best time for practising yoga asanas is in the early morning when the stomach is empty and the bowels have been emptied. If you are going to practise at any other time during the day make sure that you do not practise on a full stomach. This is dangerous. Allow at least three or four hours after a full meal and one hour after a snack meal.

3. Yoga asanas are best done on the floor — not on a bed, however firm. On a thick carpet or thin foam pad spread a clean sheet which should be kept only for yoga and which should be washed and aired frequently.

4. Choose a place which is airy, quiet and free from all disturbances. Turn off the radio and television and make sure you are not disturbed by the telephone or door bell.

5. If your hair is long, tie it back. Do not wear belts or scarves.

6. Practise every single day. Without this discipline you will not be successful.

2

THE YOGA DIET

Diet plays a very important role in the successful practice of Yoga. There is a saying, 'The healthy man satisfies his hunger when he eats — the sick man satisfies his appetite.' It is true that more people become sick by wrong eating habits and a faulty diet than from any other cause. Simple, natural foods, eaten as fresh as possible and in moderation and combined with exercise and deep breathing, are the foundations for good health.

The ancient Rishis laid down with great exactness the diet which the Yogi should follow to keep vigorous, youthful and healthy. Food that was too rich and abundant, consisting of many different dishes, led to obesity, sluggishness and a dulled mind. Food that was stale, coarse, highly spiced and containing much animal flesh led to sickness and premature old age. Food that was fresh, light, wholesome and nourishing, eaten only in sufficient quantities to satisfy one's hunger but not one's appetite, was a diet that kept one forever young, forever full of energy, and ready for the higher practices of spiritual yoga.

Yogis are generally lacto-vegetarians, eating nuts, fruits, vegetables, grains and dairy products such as milk, cheese, butter, and eggs. Some Yogis (generally those who live alone in caves or in ashrams) do not eat any animal by-products, not even honey or milk, since bees are deprived of their food and often of their lives when harvesting honey, and the young animal is deprived of its rightful food when milk is taken for human consumption.

None of these rules, however, are for those who practise yoga for one hour a day. All that is necessary is moderation in all things, and a diet that is made up of fifty per cent of raw, fresh foods. Meat, especially red meat, should be reduced in the diet since it is very rich in animal fat and protein and research in Britain and the US indicate that some forms of cancer are aggravated by it. Dr Alan

Long, writing in *New Scientist*, says that a vegetarian diet need not be deficient in essential proteins if nuts, beans, legumes, pulses and grains are used. Four out of five cases of food poisioning in Britain are traced to the consumption of meat and its products.

There are many advantages to a vegetarian diet. Plant oils are generally unsaturated fats, while animal fats have a high level of triglycerides which raises the blood cholesterol level. Vegetarians get more fibre in their diet and therefore suffer much less from constipation and colonic disease. Fibre reduces the time that food takes to pass out of the body, lessening the toxins produced by bacteria which remain in the gut in non-vegetarians for a much longer time, giving rise to diverticular disease as well as cancer of the large intestine and rectum.

Whichever diet you choose, once you embark on your yoga rejuvenation programme, do not eat more than three to four ounces (100 grammes) of meat per day. Meat, eggs, fish and poultry must all be eaten very fresh if putrefactive bacilli are not to invade the large intestine in their billions and poison the system. Better still, alternate vegetarian and non-vegetarian days. As your yoga *sadhana* (training) progresses you may give up eating flesh of your own accord. Meanwhile there are certain basic rules which must be followed.

Diet for rejuvenation

1. Fifty per cent of your food should be eaten raw. Examples include vegetables, fruits, nuts, seeds, sprouted grains, yogurt, and dried fruits, as well as fresh vegetable and fruit juices.
2. Drink at least eight glasses of pure water a day. Do not drink with meals as this dilutes the digestive juices. Drink half an hour before or after a meal.
3. Eat always in moderation and slightly less than one's fill. Over-eating damages the body, reduces efficiency and makes one fat. Instead of a light, springy step, the person who eats too much drags his extra weight around or plods along heavily. He has extra bulges and protrusions all over his body instead of a slim (even lean) and shapely body.
4. Masticate your food very thoroughly. This is one rule which many people disregard. Food should be thor-

oughly chewed until it is a paste in the mouth. This has two benefits. You tend to eat less since the appetite is satisfied quicker, and your digestion improves one hundred fold. Dr Phulgendra Sinha claims that people who are overweight almost always eat very fast.

5.   Meals should be eaten in a calm and placid frame of mind, not when angry, tired or worried. Concentration should be toward the good that the food is doing, nourishing and giving us strength.

6.   Cut out all white sugar, and white flour products from your diet. Both these are not only 'empty calories', they are actually harmful and degenerating foods that clog the body, impede blood circulation and lead to all kinds of diseases.

7.   Do not salt your food at the table. Use salt very sparingly in cooking and none at all at the table. Use sea salt if possible.

8.   Avoid canned, processed foods and those foods that have additives, chemical preservatives or stabilizers. These are all dead foods and do nothing to nourish the body.

9.   Every day try to include some form of fresh sprouted grains or seeds in your diet. The importance of this will be explained later on.

10. Do not over-cook the fifty per cent of your food that is not eaten raw. Steam, broil, or stir-fry your food the Chinese way. Over-cooking kills all the vitamins and nutrients in your food. Save the water (for soups and lentils) in which you have soaked your grains or seeds for sprouting.

Scientific studies have clearly shown that there are definite links between mineral-rich, naturally fertilized soils, fresh vegetables and fruits grown in these soils and the health and emotional well-being of all human beings. Such harmonious inter-relationship of man and his surroundings ensures excellent physical health, mental stability and superior resistance to disease. It promotes healthy skin, thick glossy hair, strong, resilient muscles and good physical structure. Physical degeneration, emotional traumas, and infectious and degenerative diseases do not exist when a diet of fresh natural foods is accompanied by a yoga regime of exercise, breathing and relaxation.

A bad or incorrect diet may cause structural changes in the body, physical imperfections, sexual impotence, depression and mental confusion. It can also be the cause of alcoholism, hyperactivity, irritability, fatigue, and violence. Many delinquent children are being given diets high in vitamins and natural nutrients and their behavioural patterns have changed and improved amazingly. If the brain is starved of proper nutrition and is also constantly bombarded with food additives, insecticides, sugar, salt and white flour products, behaviour changes occur. In his book *Diet, Crime and Delinquency*, Alex Schause gives details of research supporting the effects of incorrect diet on crime. Children should never be fed 'junk' foods such as colas, hamburgers, ice-cream, tea, coffee and foods saturated with white sugar.

Refined white sugar can clog up the system and hinder the working of the entire organism of the body acting as a poison and creating a whole range of diseases. White sugar has an ageing effect on the body.

Most modern diets need to be supplemented with vitamins and minerals, since it is not always possible to obtain farm-fresh food grown in organic manure and without pesticides, insecticides and other harmful sprays.

Since old age often involves having fragile bones, so brittle that they are constantly in danger of breaking at the slightest bump or fall, care should be taken to get an adequate supply of calcium in the diet. Technically one's bones should be in equally good shape at seventy as they were at twenty and if properly nourished they can remain strong instead of degenerating into fragile sticks. Calcium is necessary for the health of every cell and if these cells do not get it from your food, they will take it from the bones, producing what is known as osteoporosis.

After the menopause women are specially vulnerable to this leaching of calcium from the bones. A jerk, or even a sudden, quick movement can cause a bone to fracture or splinter. A broken hip may mean months of being in bed till it heals. Any one older than forty should get a high calcium supply in the diet, either by supplements or from a diet rich in this substance. Green vegetables, hulled sunflower seeds, whole sesame seeds, cheese (Parmesan has the highest amount) and sardines, yogurt, wholewheat, egg yolk, dried apricots, dates and raisins as well as milk are all good sources of calcium.

Biological age is not necessarily equal to linear age and many young people, according to Dr Swami Gitananda, 'have the bodies of eighty-year-old senile degenerates, having misused their bodies so early in life. The processes of yoga and especially those of *Kaya Kalpa* will totally create a new body.'

Kaya Kalpa means body rejuvenation and part of the process is to consume as high as eighty per cent raw food. Milk and milk products, cheese and eggs are eliminated from the diet and replaced by soya milk, yogurt and wheat milk products. The whole process can only be carried out in an ashram where the yoga life is followed for twenty-four hours per day for at least six months. Modified kaya kalpa practices can, however, be successfully carried out by anyone who will change their eating habits, give up smoking and alcohol and all forms of drugs and practice yoga asanas, relaxation and breathing on a regular basis.

Foods to include in the yoga diet

Yogurt and cottage cheese
In India, yogurt is served with every meal. It is an excellent source of nourishment and provides the stomach with necessary and helpful baccilli to promote digestion, keeping the good bacterial count in the colon high. It promotes virility and prolongs life and the calcium in the fermented milk is very easily absorbed and digested. Do not use yogurt with sugar, jams, jellies or sweetened fruits. Honey may be used in small quantities. It is delicious made into *raitas* and eaten with grated cucumbers stirred in, chopped tomatoes, diced, boiled potatoes, cubed bananas or chopped herbs. It is easily made at home and here is a very simple method:

Bring milk to the boil, pour into a pottery or earthenware bowl and allow to cool to lukewarm. Stir in one teaspoon (5 ml) of yogurt to every pint (570 ml, 20 fl oz, 2½ cupsful) of milk. Cover the bowl tightly and put in a warm place such as a cooling oven. Leave over night. In the morning the yogurt will have

set firm. Chill it in the refrigerator and it will firm up
even more.

Pulses
Pulses have a very low fat content and whatever fat there
is will be polyunsaturated. All pulses are rich in protein
and if sprouted make delicious vegetable and salads, full
of Vitamin C and alpha-linolenic acid.

Wheat germ
This is one of the richest sources of the Vitamin B group. It
also includes Vitamins E and PP as well as protein, fat and
iron. Use the oil in salads and sprinkle the wheat germ on
cereals, or in soups and sandwiches. This energy-giving
food is a must for nerves and vitality.

Nuts
Everyone, and specially vegetarians, should eat a handful
of hard-shelled nuts every day. Almonds, pecans,
cashews, brazil nuts and walnuts are all excellent sources
of protein and essential fatty acids.

Sunflower seeds
These make delicious snacks and are full of nutrition. One
cup of seeds gives you the B- complex vitamins: 7 to 8 mg
of niacin, 2.84 mg of thiamine and .33 mg of riboflavin.
The seeds are rich in calcium, magnesium, iron and
potassium. 4 oz (1 cupful) of the seeds contain 920 mg of
potassium as compared with 370 mg in bananas. If
sunflower seeds are sprouted the Vitamin C value increases greatly.

Citrus fruits
Drink the juice and eat the pulp of a whole fruit every day.
An excellent source of the vital Vitamin C which promotes
healing, citrus fruit cuts through mucous and tissue
inflammation and helps alleviate respiratory infection. An
abundant supply of this Vitamin is necessary for maintaining and rebuilding muscles and body tissue. Orange,
lemon, lime, grapefruit and tomato all have these great
curative and healing properties. Lemons in particular have
large quantities of Vitamin C and they also have Vitamin
PP which protects the vascular system. They contain

traces of iron, silica, phosphorous magnesium and copper. Drink the juice of a fresh lemon in water every single day of your life to fight off indigestion and headaches caused by malfunctioning of the liver. Lemon juice helps to relieve nausea and sickness. If you are trying to lose weight, drink the juice of a small lemon, diluted in water, after every meal. If you are suffering from lumbago, sciatica or pains in the joints, grate the skin of a whole lemon, mix it with a little honey and eat it every day.

Onions and garlic

Both onions and garlic prevent germs and viral infections. One of the finest tonics for all-over health and vitality is to stir half a teaspoon of garlic juice and half a teaspoon of onion juice into a glass of warm water. Add a few drops of lemon juice and drink first thing in the morning. To expel worms, take a dose of chopped garlic mixed with a little butter and honey before going to bed at night. For a clear skin, low cholesterol, a strong heart and good digestion, eat a little chopped garlic in salad or with bread every day. Onions chopped in vinegar make an excellent appetizer and stimulate digestion. A little salt, black pepper and cummin make it good enough for a gourmet.

Honey

All those who wish to follow a rejuvenating diet must give up white sugar in all its forms. Instead, use raw honey, maple syrup or molasses. Honey is a wonderful source of energy. It calms the nerves, regulates bowel movements and cures constipation. Taken in warm milk at bedtime it is a soporific, especially if accompanied by three or four tablets of calcium. Almonds and honey are a good combination for rejuvenation and for preserving youthful vitality. Soak ten almonds in warm water overnight, and in the morning slip off the skins. Chop the almonds roughly, mix with two teaspoons of honey and eat. Within one week you will notice the difference in your vitality.

Fresh fruit and vegetables

Eat plenty of fresh fruits in season and vegetables of all kinds, especially green vegetables, the greener the better. Examples include spinach, kale, lettuce, green beans, green pepper, spring onions, brussels sprouts, cabbage and parsley. Carrots are a wonderful food and they can be munched raw, or used in salads chopped or grated, or put into the blender to make a cup of delicious vitamin-enriched juice. Eat as much of the whole fruit, skin and all, as possible. If vegetables are to be cooked, steam, broil or stir-fry them the Chinese way.

Dates, raisins, and other dried fruits
Dates are often used in aryuvedic medicine as sexual stimulants and to regain lost potency. Soak five or six dates overnight in a cup of milk. Next morning stone the dates, eat them and drink the milk. Basic sexual energy is regained, especially if combined with the honey and almond routine given earlier. All dried fruits are full of health-giving nutrition and make excellent desserts or snacks, more so if combined with some crunchy nuts. They supply a healthy form of sugar, contain some of the B complex vitamins, iron and calcium and some minerals. They are excellent for stubborn constipation. Prunes or figs should be soaked overnight in a little water and first thing in the morning, the water should be drunk and the fruit eaten.

Fats and oils
The first thing to do is to cut down on all animal fats: eat butter infrequently or just a scraping on bread or toast. Cream should only be indulged in rarely. Food should be cooked in small quantities of sunflower, soybean, cotton seed or nut oils. Avoid blends and coconut oil. The best way to use these oils is uncooked in salad dressings. Linseeds, sunflower seeds and sesame seeds are rich in beneficial oils and linoleic acid; they can be made into delicious spreads and nut butters.

Soya
This is a very rich source of protein and also contains generous quantities of mineral salts and the B Vitamins as well as Vitamins E and K. If you are tired, nervous, anaemic or depressed, eat some soya every day as a powerful regenerating food. Ground into flour, cooked as beans or as a milk substitute, soya protein is one of the most balanced and complete foods you can eat. The beans have a high percentage of fibre — ⅓ ounce (10 grms) to a

cup of beans — and are one of the best sources of lecithin, an emulsifying agent which dissolves cholesterol deposits.

Beansprouts
This is the wonder food of outstanding nutritional value, although it has only recently been recognized as such in the West. Sprouting is done from seeds or beans that are germinated indoors without the use of soil. The seeds or beans are soaked in water overnight or until they swell, then rinsed and allowed to drain. There are several ways to grow beansprouts but many journals make the whole thing seem unneccessarily complicated.

An example of how easy it is to grow sprouts happened to me as I came home in the car after a visit to the grocers. The paper bag in which I was carrying mung beans split and a handful or so of the beans spilled over the car floor. Next day the car went for servicing and the mats were swished over with water. One week later, we discovered to our astonishment, several long white sprouts, about eight inches long, sticking up from the floor of the car. Warm, damp and in the dark, the seeds had sprouted and were growing — they even had two little green leaves on each end. So don't worry about how difficult it is to grow them! After soaking and straining, spread the beans on clean paper towels, not too thickly. Cover with towels or a thick cloth which has been soaked in warm water and wrung out. Two or three times a day sprinkle with water or wring out cloth again and re-cover. In 24 hours there will be little white sprouts and the beans are ready to eat. Or if you prefer you can grow them till they are ½ inch (8mm) long which will take about three days.

All seeds and grains to be sprouted should be raw and untreated. The ones most used are legumes (beans, peas, lentils, alfalfa, fenugreek), grains (wheat, oats, rye) and members of the cabbage family (mustard, cress, radish). Remember that during germination the seeds should never be allowed to go dry. For quick germination and better flavour the temperature should be between 70° and 80°F (21° to 27°C). Airing cupboards may be used. Taste the sprouted beans at different stages to find out how you like them best. If you want the beansprouts slightly green, expose them for a few hours to indirect sunlight. Toss them in salads, sprinkle them over cooked vegetables, use them in sandwiches or in omelettes and scrambled eggs. Stir them into yogurt and flavour lightly with sea salt.

While the seeds are germinating, complex and beneficial changes are taking place. Amino acids are more digestible; the protein content increases and the fat and carbohydrates decrease. Whole wheat when sprouted is particularly good since the natural hormones released are easily absorbed and aid in rejuvenation.

All through the winter, when fresh vegetables are both expensive and hard to come by, sprouts can be safely and easily grown in your own kitchen. Niacin and Vitamin C are increased four times by sprouting. These little marvels contain Vitamin A, B-complex, C, D, E, G and K.

Perhaps you are asking yourself if all this is worth it? Can food really make all that difference? Isn't the diet I have been eating good enough? The fact remains however, that if you don't eat properly you will become sick. Heart attacks, arthritis, digestive and colonic problems, obesity, liver damage, diabetes and even cancer can be caused by faulty eating habits. You may be eating a great deal — perhaps too much — and still be starving from the nutritional point of view. The smooth, normal functioning of any part of the body depends on sufficient quantities of vitamins, minerals and other substances extracted from food.

The fasting diet
Once a year a 7-day fasting diet should be undertaken. This does not mean a total fast from all food but simply a diet in which no solids are eaten. For the first three days the diet should consist of only diluted fruit juice or a potassium broth*. For the next three days the diet should consist of fresh fruits and fresh raw vegetables, puréed, sliced or pulverized. A little honey may be used as a sweetener but absolutely no refined products. Fluid intake should be high: a minimum of eight glasses of water per day. On the last day, lightly steamed vegetables may be eaten for lunch and dinner. No milk, tea, coffee or alcohol should be taken during these seven days. Herbal teas are permitted.

At the end of the fast the body will feel light and

*See recipe given at the end of this chapter.

refreshed. Toxins will have been eliminated and there will be a definite weight loss. The skin, hair and eyes will all look and feel much better. In fact one eye doctor claims that after a total fast for two to three days many of his patients who had barely been able to see anything without their spectacles, were able to read fine print.

Menu for maximum vitality
Choose 2 or 3 items from the foods given here for each meal.

Breakfast
Fresh fruit; Juicy-Fruity breakfast*; Whole wheat bread* with cottage cheese; a glass of fruit juice, diluted; Sprouted Wheat drink*; Sprouted Wheat Breakfast*; Granola with dried fruit; 1 cup yogurt with fruit and honey; a poached or scrambled egg; oatmeal with a little fresh cream.

Lunch
Nutty meat loaf*; Vegetable and sprout salad; Eggplant with Cheese*; Green rice* with potassium broth; broiled liver with tomatoes; fish baked or broiled; Crunchy fruit and nut salad; Baked Zucchini*; cottage cheese with fruit; lentils with sprouted mung; soya bean patties.

Dinner
Cream-of-lentil soup*; stuffed peppers; steamed fish; herbed corn baked in tomato- cups*; Cheesy salad bowl; sprout and vegetable salad*; Spaghetti Parmesan*; oniony scrambled eggs*; cucumber raita*.

Snacks
Wholemeal (wholewheat) bread with cream cheese sprinkled with sprouts; Nutrition-high biscuits*; walnut-coconut biscuits*; vegetable sticks; nuts and dried fruit; any kind of fresh fruit; glass of orange, pineapple or lemon juice, diluted with water.

For optimum health, additional vitamins should be taken as well as Brewers Yeast and Bran. Mineral and vitamin supplements can prevent senility and the ageing process is retarded. For instance cell loss can occur due to the accumulation of lipofuscin known as the 'ageing pigment' which can choke nerve cells and cause a drastic loss of brain function. Vitamin E has been shown to reduce the incidence of lipofuscin in the brain by as much as forty per cent. Dr Gunther Eickham of the National Institute of Ageing says: 'For the billions of short-lived cells in our bodies to reproduce themselves they must divide. Exact replication of a cell results only when every nutrient is present in the parent in the right amount.'

Vitamins are chemical substances which bring about subtle changes in our body. We need varying amounts depending on age, weight, life-style, etc. Often vitamins are inter-dependent on each other and act with other vitamins or foods. Allergies, insomnia, depression, fatigue, osteoporosis, and a low resistance to infection are just a few symptoms of vitamin deficiency. Minerals are just as important and act in conjunction with each other and with vitamins, proteins, carbohydrates, oils and fats to help maintain good health.

Nutritional therapy is part of the yoga life-style and should be followed for best results. It has been found in ashrams that such diseases and conditions as diabetes, arteriosclerosis, high blood pressure and digestive diseases respond extremely well to a nutritional approach and natural therapy, without recourse to any drugs at all.

In most ashrams in India, however, no flesh foods are served and often even eggs are taboo, so that the western student must adjust to a totally different diet during his stay there — which could be anything from three weeks to six months or a year. The benefits are extraordinary.

Switch over **now** to a new way of eating; switch over to good nutrition for more pep and energy, smoother skin, lustrous hair, bright eyes and trimmer bodies. You will also have fewer colds, sleep better, suffer from less tension and depression and be holistically healthy. How we eat, exercise and relax largely determines whether we enjoy the days we live or suffer through them. The choice is up to you.

Recipes

Nutty meat loaf

> ¼ *cupful ground walnuts*
> ¼ *cupful ground sunflower seeds*
> ¼ *cupful ground pecans*
> ¼ *cupful ground Brazil nuts*
> 1 *chopped onion*
> 2 *beaten eggs*
> ½ *cupful cooked brown rice*
> 1 *cupful wholemeal bread crumbs*
> 1 *tablespoonful chopped olives*
> *Sea salt*
> *Freshly ground black pepper*

1.   Mix all the ingredients well in a large bowl.

2.   Pack into a lightly greased loaf pan.

3.   Bake at 375°F/190°C (Gas Mark 5) for 30 minutes.

4.   Serve with tomato or cheese sauce.

Note: This tastes remarkably like a meat loaf and is packed with nutrition.

Aubergine (eggplant) with cheese

> 1 *large (1 lb/455g) aubergine*
> *Oil*
> 1 *onion*
> 2 *large green peppers*
> 1 *small tin baked beans in tomato sauce*
> 1 *teaspoonful oregano*
> 1 *cupful grated cheese*
> *Butter*

1.   Cut the aubergine into thick slices and sauté lightly in a little oil till soft. Keep aside.

2.   Chop the onion, slice the peppers and sauté in the same oil till soft.

3.   In a large bowl, mash the baked beans and add onions, pepper and oregano. Mix together well.

4. Line a lightly oiled baking dish with a layer of aubergine slices. Cover with all of the beans and onion mixture, and sprinkle with half the cheese. Top with the rest of the aubergine slices, dot with butter and sprinkle with remaining cheese.

5. Bake at 425°F/220°C (Gas Mark 7) until bubbly.

Note: This is excellent with wholemeal bread and butter and a good crunchy salad.

Vegetable and Beansprout salad

1 *cupful thinly sliced cabbage*
2 *large grated carrots*
1 *grated apple with skin*
1 *thinly sliced onion*
1 *large green pepper, sliced thinly*
1 *cupful alfalfa or mung bean sprouts*

1. Mix all the vegetables and add any dressing preferred.

2. Serve, topped with bean sprouts.

Note: This salad can be varied infinitely by adding nuts, seeds, beets, radishes, grated turnip, cucumber or anything in season.

Baked courgettes (zucchini)

2 cupsful courgettes (zucchini), sliced with the skins
1 onion, sliced
Seasoning to taste
1 cupful grated sharp cheese
2 large eggs
½ cupful milk
1 tablespoonful tomato purée

1.   Line a greased flat baking dish with courgettes

2.   Cover with onion slices, seasoning and some grated cheese. Continue layers until dish is full.

3.   Beat eggs with milk, stir in tomato purée and pour over the top. Sprinkle with the remaining cheese.

4.   Bake at 350°F/180°C (Gas Mark 4) until the vegetables are tender and the custard is firm.

Potassium broth

4 large carrots
1 head celery with leaves
½ cupful spinach
1 large onion
4 tomatoes
1 large potato with skin
½ cupful parsley
1 ⅔ pint (930ml) water
Marmite

1.   Clean and chop carrots, celery, spinach, onion, tomatoes, potato. Wash and divide parsley into sprigs.

2.   Add vegetables to water, cover and simmer for 30 minutes.

3.   Strain, add a little marmite, and serve.

Note: This is excellent for a fasting diet or as the main dish for a light supper.

Cream of lentil soup

1 cupful dried red lentils
1 ⅔ pints water
1 chopped onion
2 cloves garlic, minced
1 carrot, diced
1 stick celery, chopped
¼ teaspoonful dry mustard
1 cupful single (light) cream
Sea salt and ground black pepper to taste

1. Wash lentils and soak overnight in water. Without draining, add vegetables and mustard. Cover and simmer for 2 hours or until lentils are very tender.

2. Blend lentils and vegetables till smooth, or force through sieve.

3. Heat thoroughly and stir in cream and seasoning before serving.

Note: This is a very hearty, filling soup — a meal in itself, if accompanied by wholemeal (wholewheat) bread and butter.

Green rice

2 cupsful cooked brown rice
½ cupful sour cream
½ cupful chopped parsley
Dash cayenne

1. Heat rice with sour cream, parsley and cayenne.

2. Serve with Creole Stuffed Peppers.

Creole stuffed peppers

1 *chopped onion*
Oil
2 *cloves garlic, minced*
2 *tablespoonsful chopped parsley*
1 *tomato, chopped*
2 *hard-boiled eggs, chopped*
½ *cupful wholemeal (wholewheat) breadcrumbs*
2 *large green peppers*

1. Sauté the onion in a little oil. Add minced garlic, parsley, tomatoes, chopped eggs and breadcrumbs and stir until well mixed. Cool.

2. Stuff peppers and place in large shallow baking dish. Drizzle with oil.

3. Cover and bake at 375°F/190°C (Gas Mark 5) for 30 minutes.

Pickled beets

3 *lbs (1.36 kilos) beets*
2 *cupsful cider vinegar*
½ *cupful honey*
½ *cupful water*
1 *stick cinnamon*
8 *cloves*
¼ *teaspoonful grated nutmeg*

1. Steam or pressure cook beets until tender. Cool and slip off skins. Slice.

2. Heat rest of ingredients together, add beets and boil for 15 minutes.

3. Spoon into jars and seal.

4. Eat after two weeks.

Cucumber raita

1 *cupful thick yogurt*
1 *cupful grated cucumber with skin*
Pinch of sea salt
1 *teaspoonful ground cummin*

1. Beat yogurt with fork till very smooth. Stir in cucumber and salt.

2. Sprinkle top with cayenne and cummin.

3. Chill and serve instead of a salad.

Note: In India, raita is made with mint, chopped cooked potatoes, chopped onions or any other vegetable. It is eaten with every meal.

Sprouted wheat breakfast

1 cupful wheat
Water
Raisins
1 dessertspoonful honey
1 teaspoonful lemon juice
A few chopped nuts
Optional: dates, figs, dried apricots

1. Soak 1 cupful of washed wheat in sufficient water to allow for swelling. Cover and leave overnight.

2. Drain and reserve water. Blend wheat with a little water for 30 seconds.

3. Add raisins, honey, lemon juice and any optional dried fruit. Dust with nuts. Serve.

Note: This is really a gourmet breakfast, high in nutrition. If you prefer, the wheat may be left for a further twenty-four hours for little sprouts to appear. This has all the wheat germ intact and a high content of the Vitamin B complex and lactic acid. The ferment changes the viscosity of bowel movements and improves intestinal flora. The honey, lemon juice and dried fruits provide a whole battery of vitamins and minerals to protect you from colds and start you off well for the day. Do not add milk to this breakfast.

Delicious wholemeal (wholewheat) bread

1 tablespoonful dried yeast granules
3 cupsful warm water
5 cupsful stone-ground wholemeal (wholewheat) flour
1 level dessertspoonful sea salt
1 teaspoonful raw cane sugar
2 teaspoonsful honey
¼ cupful oil

1.   Mix yeast in a bowl with the sugar, pour some of the warm water over it, stir in and allow to stand until the mixture goes frothy.

2.   Put all the dry ingredients in a bowl, make a well in the centre and pour in the yeast liquid, the honey and the oil. Stir with a wooden spoon and gradually add the rest of the warm water.

3.   Divide the dough into two and knead and turn until it is smooth and elastic.

4.   Place into two buttered tins and allow to rise until high, for about fifteen minutes.

5.   Bake at 500°F/250°C (Gas Mark 9) for 35 — 40 minutes. The loaves will sound firm if tapped on the bottom. Cool, wrap and store in refrigerator.

Note: This bread has a very smooth texture and is simply delicious to eat.

Juicy fruity breakfast

1 cupful oats, rolled
1 cupful orange juice
Honey if required
3 cupsful cut up fresh fruit, e.g. bananas, apples, peaches, pears,
Any berries, plums, pineapple
½ cupful nuts
Double (heavy) cream

1. Mix oats with orange juice, honey, fruit and nuts.

2. Soak for one hour. Eat with a little whipped cream.

Walnut-coconut bars

2 whole eggs
½ cupful honey
½ cupful wholemeal flour
¼ teaspoonful sea salt
1 teaspoonful baking powder
½ cupful grated coconut
1 cupful finely chopped walnuts

1. Separate egg yolks and beat with honey by electric beater until thick.

2. Sift flour, salt and baking powder into a bowl.

3. Stir in coconut, and nuts and then add egg yolks and honey.

4. Beat egg whites until stiff peaks form, and stir this lightly into the mixture.

5. Pour into greased and lined baking tin and bake at 350°F/180°C (Gas Mark 4) for 30 minutes until firm. Cut into bars when cold.

Nutrition-high biscuits

> 1 cupful wholemeal (wholewheat) flour
> ¼ cupful soya (soy) flour
> ¼ cupful wheat germ
> Pinch of sea salt
> 1 teaspoonful baking powder
> 2 tablespoonsful vegetable oil
> ¼ cupful yogurt
> ¼ cupful nuts
> ¼ cupful raisins

1.   Mix together wheat and soya flours and wheat germ.

2.   Add sea salt and baking powder, and stir in oil and yogurt.

3.   Knead lightly to mix. Add nuts and raisins and knead again.

4.   Drop using teaspoons onto a buttered baking tray.

5.   Bake at 375°F/190°C (Gas Mark 5) for 10 minutes.

Note: These can be served warm for breakfast.

Fruit and nut salad

> Any fruits in season — e.g. apples (with skins), orange sections, bananas, melon balls, papaya, pineapple
> ¼ cupful chopped almonds
> 1 tablespoonful orange juice
> 1 tablespoonful honey

1.   Mix cut up fruits and nuts in a glass bowl.

2.   Pour orange juice and honey over fruit.

3.   Allow to stand for some time and serve as delicious dessert.

Sprouted wheat drink

1 cupful yogurt
½ cupful wheat sprouts
1 cupful orange juice
1 teaspoonful Brewer's Yeast
1 teaspoonsful honey

1.   Put all ingredients into the blender with some crushed ice and blend until frothy.

Note: This makes a good mid-morning snack to fight off hunger pangs or tiredness.

Granola with dried fruit

1 cupful flaked oats
½ cupful wheat berries
½ cupful soya grits
1 cupful brown rice
2 tablespoonsful safflower or olive oil
½ cupful honey
1 cupful mixed chopped nuts
½ cupful sunflower seeds
½ cupful sesame seeds
1 cupful mixed chopped dried fruit

1.   Mix all grains in a bowl and pour in oil and honey. Stir to coat grains well.

2.   Bake at 350°F/180°C (Gas Mark 4), stirring every few minutes until grains are well toasted but not burnt.

3.   Cool slightly, break into chunks and stir in nuts, sunflower and sesame seeds, dried fruit and raisins.

4.   Store in air-tight tins or jars in a cool, dry place.

Oniony scrambled eggs

6 eggs
2 tablespoonsful butter
½ cupful chopped green onions
2 tablespoonsful milk
Sea salt and ground black pepper

1.   Beat all ingredients together, including unmelted butter.

2.   Stir over a low heat until on the point of setting.

3.   Remove from heat and continue to stir till set.

Spaghetti parmesan

8 oz (225 g) wholemeal spaghetti
4 cloves garlic, minced
¼ cupful olive oil
1 cupful grated Parmesan cheese

1.   Cook spaghetti in boiling salted water till just done. Drain.

2.   Add the oil, garlic and parmesan. Toss and serve hot.

Herbed corn in tomato cups

1 chopped onion
Oil
2 cupsful corn
Sea salt and ground black pepper
½ cupful minced fresh herbs (parsley, thyme, basil or savory)
4 large tomatoes

1. Cook onion in a little oil until soft. Add corn, seasoning and herbs.

2. Scoop out centres of tomatoes and fill with corn mixture.

3. Bake at 350°F/180°C (Gas Mark 4) for 30 minutes in a shallow baking dish.

Note: Serve with salad and wholemeal bread.

3

PRANAYAMA — BREATHING THE YOGA WAY

Pranayama is the control of the Vital Force (Prana) in the air we breathe, the Divine Energy, supporting and sustaining all functions of life. Most of this energy is received through the air we breathe, but some is also absorbed through food and water that we consume and some through the exposed nerve ends of the body.

All activities of life depend upon the processes of oxidation and reduction of carbon dioxide in the body. Without oxygen there is no life. Unfortunately the majority of us are shallow breathers; we do not take in enough oxygen to feed the brain and the blood–stream. Slow, deep and controlled yogic breathing allows us to provide enough oxygen for all our needs and to store up Prana, the life force, for great vitality and strength. Pranayama is one of the three foundations of good Hatha Yoga: the life-giving current which keeps us healthy and free from disease.

Very few people breathe deeply and fully enough to stretch the muscles of throat, chest and abdomen, and without that stretch they do not function properly. The average person breathes fifteen times a minute, using less than one-tenth of his or her breath capacity. Proper yogic breathing teaches us to slow down the rate and to fill the lungs with a good supply of oxygen, breathing out carbon dioxide so that the lungs and the circulating blood are purified.

Shallow breathing does not affect the nerve receptors which are buried deep inside the lungs, controlling the ability to breathe in and out and also the ability to hold one's breath. A body may be well-nourished and yet the blood may be 'oxygen starved'. The brain does not receive sufficient of this nutrient to function properly. Geronto-logists confirm that the ageing process of the body is caused partially by a decreased amount of oxygen sup-plied to the brain and they tell us that if oxygen is denied to the brain the result can be hallucination and senility.

How can we combat this general build-up of toxins and get rid of the carbon dioxide in the blood? Pranayama first cleanses the body and then recharges it with healing oxygen.

Ordinary breathing is largely an automatic process but in yogic breathing the whole breathing function is controlled by the conscious mind. Rejuvenation starts with correct breathing. Life is breath and when it ceases, we expire.

Yogic breathing mostly consists of three or four phases. These are:

(i)   *Puraka* — the controlled inhalation practised slowly.
(ii) *Kumbhaka* — the controlled suspension of breath after inhalation.
(iii) *Recaka* — the controlled exhalation of the breath.
(iv) *Sunyaka* — the suspension of the breath after exhalation.

While some simple pranayamas are just deep in-and-out breathing, others suspend the breath after inhalation or after exhalation or both, for various different counts.

Unless one is living in an ashram and dedicating one's entire life to the practice of yoga, there is no advantage in learning more than perhaps half a dozen or so, to promote good health, strong nerves, and a perfectly functioning internal system. For lessening tension and helping us to relax, there is nothing like deep, rhythmic breathing. Conversely, the quickest way to energize the system is also by deep rhythmic breathing.

Learning how to breathe
The basis and beginning of all yogic breathing is the three-part breathing technique which takes in air first in the abdominal area, then in the chest and lastly in the clavicular area. The breath is inhaled, low, mid, high and exhaled in the same order: low, mid, high.

Generally, men are good abdominal breathers and poor mid-chest breathers. Women, because of their physical make-up, are generally good at mid-chest breathing, although if they wear tight clothes or restricting corsets and belts, the breathing is restricted to the high clavicular area. For maximum benefits, all three types of breathing must be learnt and then put together smoothly to combine into one great yogic breath. Inhaling and exhaling is done slowly through the nose and with the mouth closed.

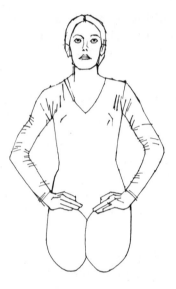

Figure 1   Vajrāsana (Diamond Posture)

Abdominal or low breathing
This form of breathing governs the flow of blood into the lower pelvis and the legs. If neglected, all sorts of negative conditions appear such as painful or irregular menstrual flow, haemmorhoids and varicose veins, oedema or water retention in the ankles, feet and knees and cold feet through bad or imperfect circulation. Blood circulation into the sacral and pelvic areas and into the legs is affected by this form of breathing.

Sit in Vajrasana (Figure 1). Keep the spine very straight and the heels well tucked under the buttocks. Put one hand on the abdominal area just below the chest. Breathe out and relax all muscles. Now inhale, filling the abdominal area with air so that the hand is pushed out as the air fills in. Breathe in and out deeply for a few rounds, feeling the hand go in and out with the breath. Now move the hands to the outer sides of the lower rib cage and breathe deeply in and out. Feel the hands expand with the ribs as the breath is inhaled and contract as the breath is let out. Breathe in and out a few times and then shift the hands around to the back and breathe into the lower back lobes, again feeling the hands move in and out with the breath. Now combine the three segments smoothly. Breathe in and inflate first the front, then the sides and then the back. Breathe out in the same way: first back, then sides and then front. For most people this is a very strange and new way to breathe and it may take a little time to get used to. Persevere. The benefits are enormous. Breathe a few times in all three lobes and then kneel up, stretch your legs and relax. Now try a special posture which forces breath automatically in the correct abdominal area, also firming up a flabby tummy at the same time.

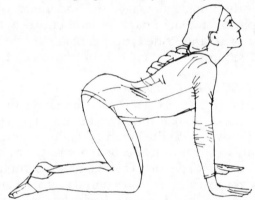

Figure 2 'In' breath-Vyaghrahāsana (Tiger Posture)

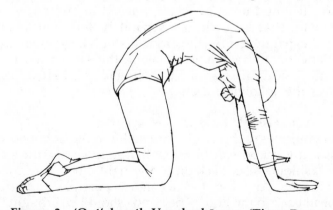

Figure 3 'Out' breath-Vyaghrahāsana (Tiger Posture)

Vyaghrahasana (The Tiger Posture) (Figure 2.)
Kneel on all fours on your yoga mat. Inhale deeply and lift

the head high and let the back hollow out so that the abdomen sags toward the floor. Hold position briefly.

Exhale (Figure 3) and arch the back as high as possible, like a big cat stretching. The stomach is pulled in and the head lowered between the arms. Stretch and hold position. Inhale and allow the abdomen to sag down while lifting head. Breathe out and arch back. Repeat these movements several times before sitting back on heels. Relax.

Benefits:
The diaphragm is considered the second heart, the source of life, the *Hara* of the Japanese. In addition to sending fresh blood into the pelvis, the sex organs and the feet, the movement of the breath massages the abdominal organs so that the spleen, stomach, pancreas and entire digestive tract is massaged and toned up. Peristaltic activity is speeded up, helping to rid the body of poisonous toxins.

Inter-Costal of Mid-Chest Breathing
Sit in Vajrasana (Figure 1). Place one hand on the area between the breasts. Exhale and then breathe in deeply so that the hand moves with the breath, pushing it out. Now place the hands on the outside of the chest, under the armpits and breathe in deeply. Feel the ribs expand like an accordion as you breathe in and contract as you breathe out. Now move the hands to the back, fingers pointing toward the spine and inhale and exhale slowly and deeply, feeling the hands being pushed in and out with the breath. Practice each lobe separately and then inhale slowly, expanding first the front of the chest, then the sides and finally the back. Exhale in the same way, first back, then sides, then front. To help mid-chest breathing, practise the following asana.

Matsyasana (Fish Posture) (Figure 4.)
Sit on your mat with your legs folded into the Lotus Pose. If this is not yet possible for you then simply cross the legs tailor fashion. Relax back on to the right elbow and then on to the left. Arch the chest as high as possible, and drop the head back to the floor. The hands should be brought to catch the toes but in the beginning you may keep the elbows to support you, on either side. In the classic position the body rests on the firm base formed by the

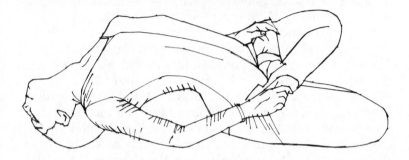

Figure 4   Matsyāsana (Fish Posture)

folded legs, and on the head. Breathe deeply and you will see that the breath comes in the mid-chest area only. Stay in this position for as long as possible, then release tension from the neck and rest it on the mat. Straighten legs, relax the hands and elbows and relax.

Benefits:
Mid-chest breathing has an excellent effect on the heart as well as the lungs. Scientific studies have shown that Matsyasana reduces high blood pressure and brings about a beneficial heart massage to build strong muscles in this area. It is the best posture in which to teach mid-chest breathing, especially for men, who find this form of breathing very difficult and who therefore have a much higher incidence of heart attacks than women. An unsatisfactory blood supply into this area can lead to constriction of blood into the pectoral muscles, causing angina and myocardial ischaemia.

Clavicular or High-Lobe breathing
This form of breathing is not a normal part of the autonomic breathing function. Very few people breathe properly in this area which remains filled with stale, oxygen-deprived air. Sometimes women who are very conscious of their figures and used to wearing tight-waisted clothes, corsets and brassières that constrict the bosom, can breathe *only* in this area: quick, shallow breaths that make them appear to be struggling for breath.

Sit in Vajrasana (Figure 1). Place one hand on the upper chest area just under the collar bones. Breathe deeply, inhaling so that the hand rises with the breath. Don't force this movement. With practice it will come naturally. Remove the hand and concentrate in the high area under the armpits. Breathe deeply, pushing this area up and out. Take your hands over your shoulders and place them on the back, on either side above the shoulders. Inhale deeply and concentrate the mind on filling these high lobes. Exhale and let them deflate. Now combine the three movements, inhaling and forcing air into the high lobes in front, then at the sides and finally at the back. Exhale in the same way: first the back, then the sides and then the front.

This is possibly the hardest of the three areas in which to breathe correctly and it may take some time before you get the hang of it. Persevere. This form of breathing is very important since it circulates blood up into the neck and head areas and into the cells of the brain, preventing loss of hearing, weakening of the eyes, headaches, tensions of all types and even loss of hair. To help force stale air from the upper lobes try *Maha Mudra*.

Maha Mudra (The Mighty Tidal Gesture)
Sit in Vajrasana (Figure 1). Keep a very straight spine and clasp the hands behind the back, pulling the hands right down so that the arms are straight. Inhale deeply and hold the breath in for a short spell. Now begin to exhale, bending slowly forward till your head rests on the mat in front of your knees. As you bend, raise the clasped hands and arms straight up into the air high toward the sky. Rest in this tense position for some time before straightening up, inhaling as you do so and bringing the hands, still locked, to their starting position behind the back. Pull the hands down toward the floor, pushing the sternum of the chest forward to expand the rib cage. Repeat this six to eight times.
Benefits:
The breath is literally moved like the tide in the ocean by this mudra. Air that has been trapped in the high lobes of the lungs will be released and stale air replaced by fresh oxygenated air. Asthmatics and those who have difficult breathing problems will find almost instantaneous relief after practising this mudra.

Now that we have learned how to breathe sectionally

we can unite all three to produce the complete yoga breath pattern.

Mahat Yoga Pranayama (The Grand Yoga Breath)
Sit in Vajrasana (Figure 1). Inhale first into the abdominal area to a slow count of three. (You may use your hands in the beginning to help identify each different area.) Now consciously shift the attention to the mid-chest area and fill this area to a slow count of three. Now move the breath up into the clavicular area, breathing in to a slow count of three. Hold breath briefly and then exhale by first releasing the air from the abdominal area, then from the mid-chest and finally from the clavicular area. Much conscious attention has to be paid in the beginning to this unfamiliar breathing pattern but it sounds more difficult than it really is. As with all yoga practices the conscious- ness must be directed, single-mindedly, to what you are doing. Only then will you reap benefits. Dr Swami Gitananda says, 'This order of breath is in complete harmony with the computer-like respiratory centre of the brain. Signals going out from that centre order the breath to come in this order. Re-establishing harmony with the breath and the computer-like respiratory centre of the brain, affords benefits that cannot possibly be described in words.'
Benefits:
Nevertheless, we will try to explain the benefits of this form of breathing which is the only proper way to breathe for perfect health and for rejuvenation. The lungs are completely filled and then emptied again. A greater supply of fresh blood is brought into the blood-stream, improving the quality of the vital organs, the endocrine glands, the nerve centres and body tissues. The brain is fed with freshly oxygenated blood. Impurities are elimin- ated and metabolism stimulated. This form of deep breathing should be practised every day — or even twice a day — for two weeks before starting on any other pranayamas. It is important to get used to this deep breathing before going on to learn more complicated forms of breathing. Many yoga teachers claim that learning just this form of breathing is enough to produce good, vital health when combined with asanas and relaxation.

Savitri Pranayama (The Rhythmic Breath)
In this breathing, inhalation and exhalation take exactly the same time, but now we add a held-in breath and a held-out breath equal to half the time of the inhaled and exhaled breath. It is very important to concentrate mentally to get used to the rhythm.

Sit in Vajarasana (Figure 1), keeping the chest, neck and head in a straight line. Rest the hands on the thighs close in to the body. Inhale slowly to the count of six, hold the breath for a count of three, exhale slowly to a count of six and hold the breath out for a count of three. Try to get a really smooth rhythm into the breathing without straining in any way. Your breath will go like this: 6x3x6x3. Repeat this several times. Feel that with each inhalation the body is being filled with calm, healing breath and with each exhalation this is being absorbed by every fibre of the body.

When you become used to this rhythm (perhaps after several days of regular practice), learn to slow down the breath even more. Now extend the breathing to a 8x4x8x4 pattern. When this is easy, slow it down further to a 10x5x10x5 and then 12x6x12x6. You will now be breathing less than twice a minute. Instead of quick, shallow breaths you are taking slow, rhythmical, deep breaths which revitalize your whole system.
Benefits:
Your life can be revolutionized by this form of breathing, which is relaxing, reviving and restoring for tired and frayed nerves or an exhausted body. Starving tissues and cells are rejuvenated. People who can't sleep will find this very soothing and even more relaxing than sleep. The face becomes relaxed, tired lines smooth out, ageing muscles are revived with fresh blood and the whole body is at peace. Dr Swami Gitananda provides this useful guide to the effects of the various rhythms.

6x3x6x3 — This is beneficial for a narrow-chested woman or an undeveloped teenager or an adult suffering from emotional swings as in manic depression. It is one of the best means of infusing Prana into the emotional body and getting control of radical emotional swings.

8x4x8x4 — This rhythm is in harmony with the cellular

vibration of the blood, muscles and skeletal structure. It is the best rhythm to strengthen and rejuvenate the body. Excellent physical health is afforded and proper electrolytic balance of the cells maintained. This is a good rhythm also for quietness and meditation.

10x5x10x5 — Metabolism is increased, speeding up the rate at which the body organs work. This is extremely beneficial for anyone with sluggish circulation and enervated motor system.

12x6x12x6 — The mind is awakened by a Pranic flow and alertness and clearness of the senses is noted. It is good for impaired sight, hearing, etc. The student wishing to develop a good retentive memory and clearness of thought should perfect this technique. Oxygen is sent to the brain.

For those who have perfected the rhythm so far, there are higher counts: 14×7 (for serenity and peace), 16×8 (for rejuvenation of the body and longevity), and further too: 18 x 9; 20 x 10, and so on. These represent breathing techniques which must be carried out under a guru's instruction, and are not advised at this stage. It is enough if you can perfect this much so that deep harmony permeates the entire body. It is one of the most important of all forms of yogic breathing and should be carried consciously into your everyday life. When you have a moment to spare, whether you are walking, sitting, or relaxing, let the rhythmic breath bring harmony and health to body and mind.

Bhastrika Pranayama (The Bellows Breath)
There are many different forms of this type of breathing but it is enough for our purpose to learn two. The breath is inhaled through the nostrils and exhaled explosively, either through mouth or nostrils.

Mukha Bhastrika (Bellows Breathing Through The Mouth)
Sit back on your heels in Vajrasana (Figure 1). Inhale slowly, a complete three-part breath, filling all three segments of the lungs. Hold the breath briefly, pucker up the lips as though you were about to whistle and then

blast the air out in short, sharp, blasts through the mouth, bending slowly forward from the waist as you do so, until your head rests on the carpet in front of your knees and all the breath has been expelled. Rest in this position before returning to a sitting position, inhaling deeply as you come up. Repeat at least twice more.

Benefits:

This is a cleansing breath, excellent for getting rid of stale air in the lungs and reducing the carbon dioxide content. It is a good pranayama to do between asanas to expel tiredness and is invigorating. Toxins are expelled and the blood cleansed. If you have been sitting in an enclosed, stuffy room and inhaling impure air, do this Bhastrika when you get home.

Narsaga Bhastrika (Bellows Breathing Through The Nose)

In this pranayama the movement of the lungs is like a bellows. Sit in Vajrasana and exhale. Now breathe in and out through the nostrils very rapidly at the rate of about two rounds per second. The abdominal area should be pushed out as you inhale and sucked in as you exhale. The movement is all in the lower abdominal area. First try it very slowly till you get the idea, then speed up the breath. Do not gasp or choke. The breath will make a smooth sssssss noise. Do ten rounds, stop, and then repeat another ten rounds. Increase the number of rounds gradually day by day, and practise twice a day.

Benefits:

This is a powerful exercise and will build strong lungs and increase your vital capacity. It relieves inflammation of the nose and throat and destroys phlegm. It is good for chronic colds and warms up the body, especially in the winter.

An extension of the Nasarga Bhastrika is to use it on any part of the body that needs healing or rejuvenating. After a few rounds of the breath, exhale and then inhale very slowly and hold the breath for as long as is possible. Now release the breath very slowly concentrating on that part of the body which needs attention. For instance, if you have a backache, slowly exhale, thinking of your back and feeling the powerful healing properties of the breath. Repeat the whole thing thrice and then curl up and relax. Do not try this on another person — it can be dangerous.

Ujjayi (Energy-renewing breath)

There are many different versions of this pranayama and different teachers seem to teach it in many ways. The distinctive feature of this, however, is that air is inhaled and exhaled through a half-closed glottis, which produces a curious sobbing sound.

Sit in any comfortable yoga position. Exhale completely. Now the glottis is partially closed and air is inhaled through both nostrils while expanding the chest. The abdominal muscles are slightly contracted throughout. The facial muscles must be relaxed and no contortions should be made. When enough air has been inhaled, the breath is exhaled slowly, again through a partially closed glottis, producing a smooth sound and the abdominal muscles are contracted more and more until the lungs are completely empty and the chest has sunk inward. Practise this breath only twice on the first day, increasing every day till ten inhalations and exhalations can be made.

Benefits:

When this pranayama is done every day it has marvellous effects. Low blood pressure is made normal, the endocrine glands are stimulated and coughs and colds become a thing of the past. The thyroid gland in particular is subjected to a strong positive current, increasing metabolism and the powers of comprehension. Elderly people with high blood pressure should not practise this breathing.

Alternate nostril breathing is given great emphasis in yoga as it is believed that when both nostrils work evenly — that is, one is not congested while the other works freely — then health is ideal. This Alternate Breathing is known as 'anulomaviloma' and there are many different variations where one nostril is closed and the other used for inhaling or exhaling. One of the best of the alternate nostril breaths is Nadi Shodhana.

Nadi Shodhana (Alternate Nostril Breathing)

Sit in Vajrasana or any comfortable yogic sitting position. Exhale completely. Although there are special hand controls for this form of breathing, in the beginning it is enough to simply use the thumb and little finger to control the breath as it comes through the nostrils.

Start the first breath by inhaling through the right

nostril. Close the nostril with the thumb and exhale through the left nostril. Suspend the breath for a brief while and inhale through the left nostril. Close the left nostril with the little finger and exhale through the right nostril. It is easy to be confused in the beginning but take it very slowly: In from the right, close nostril; out through the left, suspend breath and then in through left; close left nostril and out through the right; in right, out left, in left, out right, in right, out left, and so on. Do this breathing to the rhythmic breath that you have already learned.
Benefits:
This establishes equilibrium of the positive and negative currents in the body. It calms and strengthens the nerves, cures insomnia and stabilizes the mind. It has beneficial effects on the digestion, circulation and nervous system.

Pranava Pranayama (Vibratory Breathing)
This is a form of deep breathing done to the sound OM. It is not necessary to believe that OM is a sacred word. Simply believe that it is unique and has powerful effects when combined with deep breathing.

Sit on your yoga mat in any straight-backed position. Breathe in slowly and deeply, taking in the breath first low, then mid, then high. Now hold in the breath briefly and then exhale. As you begin the exhalation from the abdominal area, sound the 'Aah' audibly. When all the breath has been exhaled from this area begin exhaling in the mid-chest area as you sound the 'Ooooo' audibly and evenly. Then proceed to the high clavicular area and sound 'Mmmmmmm' till all the breath is exhaled. The 'Aah' is a low guttural sound, the 'Oooo' is from the chest and the 'Mmmmm' vibrates high in the head. Together the three sounds make up the sound OM or AUM. When you get used to this adjust your breath pattern so that the exhalation is twice as long as the inhalation. If you inhale to the count of four, then exhale to the count of eight. Increase the counts as you get more proficient till you can inhale to the count of ten and exhale to the count of twenty.
Benefits:
This type of breathing has powerful health benefits. The vibrations reach down to the air in the lungs stimulating the pulmonary cells and producing significant effects on

the endocrine glands. Dr Lesser-Lazario of Vienna cured himself and many of his patients by sound therapy which consisted of sounding all the vowels with the full power of the breath. He spent twenty-five years of his life in the study of the effects produced on the body by vibrations of sound. The Yogis go one step further: instead of using any sound they use what they call the 'sound of all sounds — OM' to vibrate through the body. When the sounds are accompanied by exhalation, then the vibrations massage various important organs, reaching the deep-lying tissues and nerves, and increasing the stimulation of hormones into the blood.

The Pranava Pranayama has extensive health benefits for anyone suffering from any form of disease, mental tension or nervous disabilities. The vibrating effect has a powerful effect on the entire system. The entire body relaxes under the influence of this powerful internal vibro-massage, and the cranial nerves too are benefited by the high 'Mmmmmmm' sounded into the upper chest area and finally into the head.

After you have finished several repetitions of this form of breathing, lie down with your head to the north and relax. A desire to be quiet will usually occur, while the sound AUM still vibrates noiselessly in your entire system. Powerful forces of good will surround you. Be aware of them. Lie quietly and imagine body, mind and spirit all harmoniously united in yoga union.

Do not rush while learning what is almost certainly an entirely new way to breathe. All effort and strain must be banished. Since yogic breathing is an integral part of practising the asanas, it must be learnt first. Later, in the chapter on relaxation, we will learn two more pranayamas which are part of the relaxation process. Meanwhile, practise consciously and steadily every day. You will soon see the wonderful results.

4

ASANAS — YOGIC POSTURES

In Chapter I we learnt the conditions under which asanas must be carried out. Let me add to this: please do not wear shoes while practising. Sometimes, in western magazines, models may be seen demonstrating one or the other asana *with shoes on*! This is absolutely wrong. Every asana has some sort of acupressure point for the feet which has different, beneficial effects. Socks may be worn, but not shoes of any kind.

Asanas should be performed gradually and with caution. People over the age of forty generally have stiff bodies, unused to bending and stretching. The muscles are inelastic and the spine is rigid. Do not attempt more than two asanas per day at first. You are not in competition with anyone, even yourself. Your aim is to regain a supple, youthful and healthy body, a digestive and glandular system that works perfectly and an endocrine and circulatory system that is in prime condition. If you cannot accomplish the pose as depicted in the illustrations (and this is unlikely unless you are a ballet dancer or gymnast!) do only as much as is possible for you. Gradually, as you become more supple, you will be able to complete the posture. However little you do will be of great benefit.

One of the chief characteristics of old age is stiffness. This often exists because of a lack of exercise or because of exercise of the wrong kind. Lactic acid accumulation in the muscles can also cause stiffness. Yoga minimizes lactic acid build-up while working the lungs, heart and muscles sufficiently to result in a conditioning effect. When the asanas are combined with deep, slow breathing, the oxygen supply to muscles increases and metabolic wastes are cleansed. Blood lactate levels are dramatically lowered after twenty to forty minutes of a yoga work-out. If we do not use our bodies properly there is a wasting away of muscles, tissue and bone density. *'Use it or lose it,'* say the experts. Doctors claim that an elderly person is more likely to break a bone from sitting long hours in a chair than from controlled but vigorous exercise. Osteoporosis is as much due to lack of calcium in the bones as to lack of movement.

If you are over sixty, jogging, tennis, running, and other forms of too vigorous exercises are unsuitable. Yoga is ideally suited to everyone, from children over ten years of age to people in their sixties, seventies or even eighties.

Asanas exercise the spine by bending first in one direction and then in another so that elasticicty is restored. As each posture is held for thirty seconds or more, pressure is exerted on glands, forcing them to spurt into activity.

One of the most difficult things about Yoga, it is said, is the fact that it must be practised every day. This should be the time you give to yourself as an investment in your good health. No one is too busy to devote twenty to forty minutes a day as an investment for good health and vitality. After your yoga practice there is the psychological benefit of mood elevation and stress reduction, with a general feeling of euphoria. Dr Robert Homes of the University of Washington Medical School has pointed out that stress can accumulate to cause disease. Yoga releases stress and diminishes tension. The body is charged with oxygen, the brain clear and alert and metabolism increased. If you want to lose weight, do not eat for at least half an hour after your yoga practice. As you start this programme, visualize yourself as slim, supple, full of energy, with bright eyes, glossy hair and smooth skin. At this end of this chapter, suggested asanas for those aged over sixty are given.

Sitting Postures
VAJRASANA (The Diamond Posture) (Figure 5, side view)
Technique:
Kneel on your yoga mat and sit back on your heels, keeping them well tucked in under the buttocks. The back is held very straight with head, shoulders and buttocks in a straight line. The hands may be turned palms down, on the top of the thighs. This is one of the easier sitting postures in yoga and specially suitable for Western students who find the Lotus Pose difficult, if not impossi-

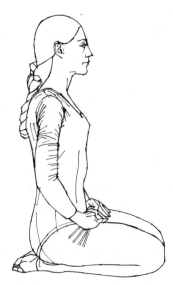

Figure 5   Vajrāsana (Diamond Posture)

ble. It is often used for all breathing exercises and also for
Zen meditation. It is not as easy as it looks and takes a
little getting used to since the ankles, feet and calves will
all ache and feel cramped in the beginning. The legs can be
eased by kneeling up, stretching and then sitting back on
the heels.

Benefits:
Vajra is a diamond but also a thunderbolt. It is an excellent
posture with which to begin a practice of yoga. It has a
good effect on the lower back and the large group of
nerves which start in the lumbar area, passing through
buttocks, thighs, knees and calves. Circulation into these
areas and into the feet is improved and severe cases of
varicose veins and haemorrhoids can be cured. It is the
only asana which can be practised directly after a meal. In
fact it is recommended for all those who suffer from
digestive disturbances. The Yogis say 'He who sits for ten
minutes in Vajrasana after eating, can digest stones.'

SIDDHASANA (Adept's Posture) (Figure 6)
Technique:
Sit on the mat with your legs straight in front. Bend the
right leg at the knee and draw the heel close to the
perineum. The leg from the knee to the heel must lie flat

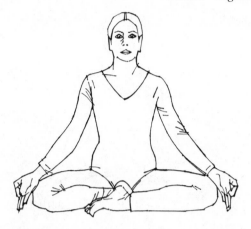

Figure 6   Siddhāsana (Adept's Posture)

along the floor. Bend the left leg at the knee and place the left leg over the right ankle or place it (as in illustration) in front of the right foot and flat on the floor. Stretch the arms out and rest the back of the hands on the knees, palms upward. Join the thumbs and forefingers together to make a circle and extend other fingers straight out.
Benefits:
This posture calms and soothes the nerves and cures stiffness of knees, ankles and thighs. It prevents rheumatism. The pelvic region is supplied with a massive supply of blood, which tones up this whole area as well as the coccyx. The body is in a calm restful position while the mind is attentive and alert. The posture may be repeated once by reversing the position of the legs.

PADMASANA (The Lotus Pose) (Figure 7)
Technique:
This is basically the meditation posture which may also be used for Pranayama. Sit on the yoga mat and place the right foot on the left thigh and the left foot on the right thigh. The feet should be far enough back to touch the heels to the abdomen on either side. The hands rest on the knees, palms open, thumb and forefinger jointed in the gesture known as 'Jnana Mudra'. The hands may also be placed one on top of the other, palms up, right hand atop the left and both hands resting just below the navel — the Buddha's favourite posture. If you can neither get your

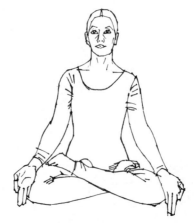

Figure 7   Padmāsana (Lotus Pose)

knees down to the floor nor cross one leg over the other, then practise at first with only one leg. As the knees and ankles become less stiff you will be able to complete the pose. There are some people however, who can do almost any asana — stand on their heads, back-bend into the wheel, do the diffcult Royal Pigeon, and yet when it comes to the Lotus Pose they have difficulty. I must add here that almost all Indians can do this easily but even here there are exceptions: one woman who went as a delegate to a yoga conference in the States, could not accomplish this pose!

Benefits:

This is supposed to be the supreme posture for meditation, one in which the positive and negative currents are in harmony; a symbol of mental purity and developed consciousness. The nervous system is calmed and breathing becomes deep and slow. The legs, knees and ankles become very supple.

BADDHAKONASANA (Bound Hand-Foot Posture) (Figure 8)
Technique:

Sit on your yoga mat with the soles of your feet flat against each other and pressed firmly together. Catch hold of your feet and pull them as close to your body as possible, right up against the groin. Straighten the shoulders and back and try and get your knees flat down on either side, as in illustration. If you have very stiff hips and the pelvic area

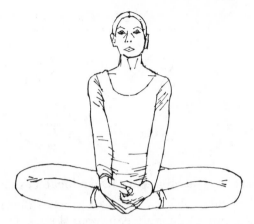

Figure 8   Baddhakonāsana (Bound Hand-Foot Posture)

is tense, this can take a long time.

You can help by 'butterflying' the knees up and down to make the hips more flexible and increase circulation in this area. If your knees stick up high on either side, press down lightly with your hands on your knees. Gradually as the knees, hips and pelvis loosen up your knees will touch down and you will be able to sit in this beautiful pose. An extension is to exhale and bend forward, touching the head down in front of the feet. Breathe deeply while in the straight sitting position.

Benefits:

This asana is extremely beneficial for both men and women who suffer from any form of urinary trouble. The abdomen and back are given a fresh supply of blood and the bladder is maintained in excellent working order. It regularizes menstrual problems and is one of the very best asanas for pregnant women who should practise it throughout the entire nine months. If you contract the anal muscles while sitting in this pose, the benefits are doubled. It is also a marvellous mood-elevator, getting rid of the 'blues' and helping to keep the mind cheerful.

DHARMIKASANA (The Devotional Pose) (Figure 9)
Technique:

This posture is also known as *Shahashasana*, the Hare posture. Sit in Vajrasana (Figure 5) and catch hold of the ankles or the feet. Exhale and bend forward until the head touches the floor in front of the knees. Be careful that you

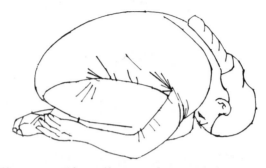

Figure 9   Dharmikāsana (Devotional Posture)

do not lift off the heels as your head touches down on the floor. Tuck your nose between your knees to get the maximum curve into the neck. Relax elbows down to the floor. Breathe normally: the breath in this position will be slow but shallow. Relax and visualize a curtain of black in front of your eyes.

Benefits:

This is a simple position (except for those who have very protruding bellies!) and has marvellous effects. The spinal cord is pulled and tugged and stretched and the cerebro-spinal fluids cushioning the spinal cord and the brain are relieved from excess pressure, so that a very deep relaxed state is attained. In experiments in Ananada Ashram in Pondicherry, Dr Swami Gitananda was able to demonstrate that the spine actually increased in length from 4 to 7 inches (10 to 18 cms) when this posture was assumed. Using stiffly knotted cords to measure the spine, first in the straight-sitting Vajrasana and then in the forward-bending Dharmikasana, there was a considerable difference — a startling difference — in the length of the spine, giving immediate, beneficial results. Localized tensions disappear, headaches are relieved, sinus problems disappear and even dizziness from car sickness is alleviated. It is an excellent posture to do between strenuous asanas, when the body is tense and needs relaxation.

VIRASANA (Hero's Posture) (Figure 10)
Technique:
This is the posture in which soldiers sat to fire off their bows and arrows. Kneel on your mat and then lift up so that you are resting on your knees and toes. The buttocks

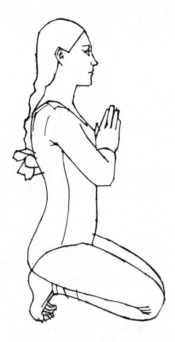

Figure 10 Virāsana (Hero's Posture)

rest on the heels. There is considerable pressure on the toes. The hands are folded into the Namaskara, the Indian gesture of greeting. From this position the hands may be raised over the head or straight in front on the inhaled breath and brought back to the original position on the exhaled breath.

Benefits:
These postures teach equilibrium and balance, strengthen the feet and toes and have the effect of releasing sexual tension and frustration. When the hands are raised over the head, Prana moves upward along the spine. In all these sitting positions flexibility of hips, legs, knees and pelvis is gained as well as a feeling of tranquillity and calmness.

Asanas for stimulating glandular activity & sexual vigour
Although these asanas are grouped under this heading they are also good to help stiffness, increase the circulation and total body health. Many asanas overlap in their effects and will be listed under two or more headings.

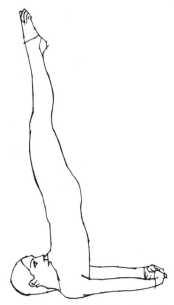

Figure 11 Sarvangāsana (Shoulder Stand)

SARVANGASANA (The Shoulder Stand) (Figure 11)
Technique:
Although this asana is known, for obvious reasons, as the Shoulder Stand, in Sanskrit it means 'all-purpose' or for the whole body. It is one of the best and most beautiful of the topsy-turvy poses and absolutely safe to do for those who cannot, or must not, practice the headstand. Lie down on your mat, arms and legs straight and the curve in the small of the back flattened out as much as possible. Take in a deep breath and lift both legs up till they are at right angles to the body. Pause and exhale. Inhale and swing legs, buttocks and lower back off the floor, supporting the back with the hands high up just under the shoulders and raising the body till it is straight and perpendicular to the floor. The chin is pressed tightly into the sternum. In the beginning if you have difficulty in attaining this position bend the knees and fold the legs against the thighs before lifting into the air. Once you are in the correct position exhale and begin to breathe deeply, keeping the breath in the abdominal area. Once you have mastered the position it should be done in one smooth movement. From the back supine position the legs are lifted smoothly, the movement continuing until the whole

body is balanced on the neck and shoulders. Hold this position with great steadiness, for a few seconds in the beginning, increasing the time every day gradually till it can be held for one minute.

Learn to come out of the Sarvangasana with great control, rolling gradually down with bent knees so that there is no flopping or crashing down on the backbone or tail bone. Relax now and do some deep breathing.
Benefits:
This posture should not be repeated more than once. The aim is to increase the time for holding. Variations are to stretch the arms down flat on the floor, or bring them up to rest on the knees, when it is known as the un-supported shoulder stand. There is hardly any area of the body which is not benefited by this asana. The chin, pressing tightly into the jugular notch, activates the thyroid glands, increasing blood supply to the whole body and speeding up metabolism. Pressure is taken off the bladder and surrounding tissues, as well as the sex organs, promoting healthier muscle cells. Since we spend so much time in the upright position this is a relief as gravity works the other way. Fresh, healthy blood circulates around the face, neck and chest, rejuvenating the skin and acting with far greater effect than all the skin creams and moisturizers on the market. Constipation and sluggishness of the bowels are cured and the abdomen is flattened as the internal organs fall into their correct places. Deep presssure is exerted on the utero-abdominal and genito-urinary organs by stretching muscles which often become relaxed with age. Since a fresh blood supply is sent to the deep muscles of the sex organs it invigorates and rejuvenates them. The Yogi Yesudian recommends that this posture is of such great benefit that everyone should practise it several times a day. It activates, according to him, not only the thyroid but also the thymus and ear glands. In this inverted position varicose veins and haemorrhoids are beneficially affected and 'long-lost youth, vital force and once-dissipated energy stream back abundantly even into the bodies of elderly people.' It is one of the best asanas to energize the body. If you are tired from working too much, simply lie down on your mat and practise the shoulder stand and feel energy flow back into every part of your body.

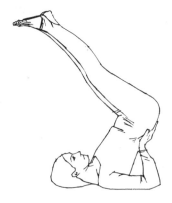

Figure 12 Viparita Karani-I (Topsy-Turvy Pose)

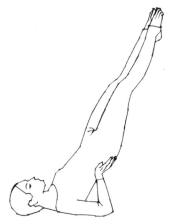

Figure 13 Viparita Karani-II (Topsy-Turvy Pose)

VIPARITA KARANI (The Topsy-Turvy Pose) (Figures 12 and 13)
Technique:
Lie on the back as for Sarvangasana. Breathe in and lift the legs and buttocks off the floor. The body is not raised straight up into the air but is only half-raised, supported by the hands on the hips, with the elbows bent and providing a firm support on the floor. Most of the weight is on the arms and elbows. The legs form an angle of roughly 70° with the ground. Breathe deeply in this position for a few seconds. Now extend the body away at an angle so that it resembles a surfboard, legs pointing out. This needs a little practice as it is a balance position

and in the beginning you may need a little help from a friend. Once you are firm and confident start the kriya or movement by fanning the legs back and forth — first over the head and then away from you and back over the head. Adjust the hands if necessary for a firmer support. Breathe in as you bring the legs over the head and out as you point them away from you. End the exercise by holding the first position with the legs forward over the head, for thirty seconds or more. Roll down slowly and relax.

Benefits:

This is the easiest of the three inverted positions which include the Shoulder Stand and the Head Stand. Almost anyone can do it. In this position the blood flows to the neck, throat and head so that the thyroid and pituitary glands are stimulated. It is often used to cure goitre. The nervous centre of the brain is regenerated and the skin of face, neck and throat are made smooth and wrinkle-free. When the legs are fanned back and forth there is a further benefit. The Islets of Langerhans within the pancreas are forced into activity, increasing the metabolism and toning up the endocrine glands. Anyone suffering from acidosis should practise this twice a day. The Islets of Langerhans secrete a hormone called insulin directly into the blood-stream to balance the sugar produced from the liver. If the pancreas does not work well, diabetes can occur. The surf-board posture, as the legs are fanned away from the body, forces the pancreas to function normally by placing extreme pressure onto this area. The gonads benefit particularly, although most of the endocrine glands are excited into activity by this backward and forward movement of the leg.

SHIRSHASANA (The Head Stand) (Figure 14)

Technique:

So much has been written about this famous pose that many of my students feel they have not learned yoga unless they can stand on their heads. As asanas go it is not particularly difficult, but it does have certain adverse effects for many people. In fact, many ashrams refuse to teach this asana unless the student has had a thorough medical examination. At the end of this section I will list the limitations for practising this posture.

Sit down on the floor in Vajrasana (Figure 5). Fold a

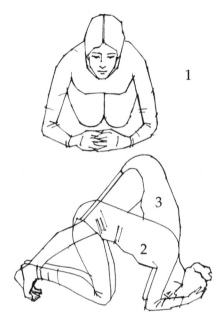

Figure 14 (1, 2 & 3) Shirshāsana (The Headstand)

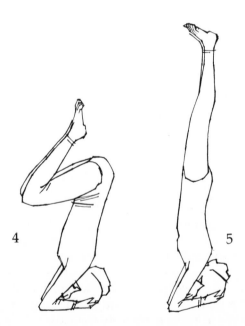

Figure 14 (4 & 5) Shirshasana (The Headstand)

blanket or sheet into four and place it on the mat in front of you. A small flat pillow will also do. Bend forward and link your fingers together, placing them on the folded blanket or pillow. The elbows are firmly placed to make a supporting triangle. The correct distance between the elbows is very important. Measure this by clenching one fist and placing it inside the opposite elbow. It should fit exactly. This will be the strong supporting tripod for the headstand. If the elbows are too far apart or too close together the balance is adversely affected. (1) shows the correct starting position.

Now place the head inside of the interlocked fingers so that it touches the floor just above the hair line, while in the kneeling position. Now walk up, straightening the knees until the back is perpendicular to the floor. The hands are still in the same position supported by the elbows. Until the body returns to the first position the hands and elbows, as well as the head, remain immovable. See Positions 2 and 3. The third position is *Makarasana* and for those who can go no further, or who are forbidden to do the complete headstand, this makes an excellent substitute. It is an inverted position: blood rushes to head and neck, the leg muscles are stretched and toned and the back exercised. There is no fear of falling and especially for those over sixty this is enough. For others it is recommended that this posture is done only for the first few days to get the feeling of being 'inverted'. If you feel the strain or tension in the neck or cracking of neck bones, then do not proceed any further.

Position 4 now begins the headstand proper. The knees are lifted on a deeply inhaled breath and pulled in close to the body. The back is straight and beautifully balanced, the toes point upward. Lean slightly back to maintain balance. When you are perfectly steady in this posture, even comfortable, we move into Position 5, the final, complete headstand. Raise the legs slowly and stretch them straight out until the whole body forms a vertical line, balanced on the head and elbows. Breathe slowly and deeply while directing the attention to the brain. Hold the position very briefly the first day, increasing gradually, a few seconds at a time, till you can stand on your head for three minutes.

To come down from the headstand bend the knees,

then the body at the hips and finally lower the legs till the feet are touching the floor and you are back to your original kneeling position. In the beginning, unless you have someone to stand beside you, do not practise in the middle of the room. You may practise against a wall by keeping your head about 3½ inches (9 cms) away from the wall. When you lift into Position 4 you will find that your back will tilt against the wall which will support you quite safely. Go into Position 5 and adjust your body so that *only the heels* are now resting against the wall. The rest of your body is in perfect alignment, balanced on the tripod of hands, elbows and head. When you are ready to practise without the help of the wall or a friend, put a thick mattress down so that if you overbalance you do not jar the spine.

Benefits:

In this asana the brain is supplied with a massive amount of fresh blood. Since every little muscle is used to maintain the balance, the body becomes supple and graceful. Pressure on the back and on the discs is relieved and weight taken off this area. If well balanced, the lumbar vertebrae in particular are placed in a most favourable position: backache caused by many hours of standing can be eliminated in a matter of seconds. Circulation into the body is reversed and the heart is relieved and filled with fresh energy. The blood drains away from the legs and the abdomen and the lungs are nourished with a pure supply of rich, oxygenated blood. The veins in the legs are able to rest, preventing varicose veins and haemmorhoids. Congestion created by long hours of sitting, which compresses the abdominal area, is cleared and relieved immediately. Prostate trouble in men, often caused by congestion, is relieved and cured by the steady practise of this asana. The genital area is also freed from congestion and the tone of this area considerably improved. Blood, which in the standing position tends to stagnate in the abdominal and pelvic area, is rapidly recirculated, improving the activity of the sex glands in both men and women. In all of the inversion postures the inner organs get a chance to return to their proper position and people with fat, flabby stomachs, will find the abdominal muscles tightening up, as everything internal begins to be pulled back, and so sagging muscles become a thing of the past. For those who want to lose weight the headstand and the yoga diet, will work together.

Limitations to the headstand

There are two schools of thought about this. Some yogis maintain that anyone, no matter how old or young, can practise the headstand safely. Others believe that the headstand is contra-indicated by several groups: by those who are over sixty and who have never practised yoga before; by those who have cervical spondilitis, since the discs in the neck are compressed and the trouble further aggravated; by those who suffer from high blood pressure; and by those who have hypertension, arteriosclerosis, heart trouble, eye troubles or kidney and liver disorders. If in doubt, practise the shoulder stand or Viparita Karani and practice a modified headstand by getting as far as Position 3, the inverted posture of *Makrasana*.

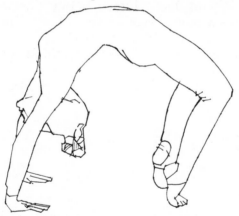

Figure 15 Chakrāsana (The Wheel)

CHAKRASANA (The Wheel) (Figure 15)
Technique:
There are two ways in which this pose may be achieved. The easier method is described first. Lie down on your yoga mat, flat on your back. Draw the heels up to the buttocks, keeping the feet slightly apart. Place the hands, palms down on the floor under the shoulders, fingers pointing towards the feet. Breathe in and lift the body off the floor until the weight is on the hands and feet and the head is lifted clear from the floor. The back is arched high and the body forms a perfect semi-circle. The more difficult method, for those who have very supple spines,

is to stand on the yoga mat, raise the arms high into the air on a deeply inhaled breath and bend back slowly, bending the knees slightly till the hands touch the floor. The body is now in the wheel position. Relax by exhaling and lying down.

Benefits:

In this beautiful pose the spine is fully articulated, giving complete mobility to the body, and fresh energy. The neck is stretched to the point of traction, which is of inestimable value to those who have any form of cervical pain and tension. The shoulders, arms, thighs, legs and trunk are all tugged and stretched. Muscle tone and spinal health is maintained by this pose and a plentiful supply of blood is fed to the nerves on either side of the spine. Calcification or deterioration of the bones, which occurs with old age when the bones become brittle, is prevented by this posture. Rheumatism, lumbago, and nerve pains are cured and the spine becomes very elastic. The abdominal muscles and the rectal muscles are activated and nourished, and obesity, constipation and congestion are remedied.

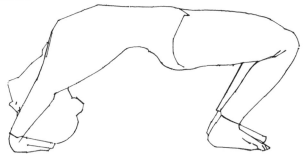

Figure 16 Vilomāsana (Inverted Posture)

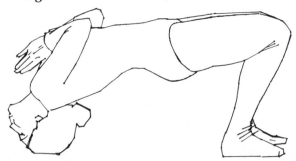

Figure 17 Vilomāsana (Inverted Posture) Variation

VILOMASANA (The Inverted Posture) (Figures 16 and 17)
Technique:
For those who find the Wheel impossible, this asana is a modified version, with almost all of the good benefits provided by the Wheel. Lie down on your back. Place your hands, fingers pointing towards feet, under your shoulders. Bend knees and pull the heels close up to the buttocks. Keep the heels about six inches (15 cms) apart. Inhale and lift the body on to the head, hands and feet. The head is tilted far back, elbows point upward toward the sky (see Figure 16). Hold position with deep breathing for ten to twenty seconds then relax the head and slide feet back to starting position. An extension of this pose, also known as *The Japanese Bridge*, is to remove the supporting hands when in position and fold them at the chest into Manaskara Mudra, the Indian gesture of greeting. Now the body rests only on head and feet.
Benefits:
This posture has many of the benefits of the Wheel. It has an excellent effect upon the muscles which are toned and invigorated. The neck is at a radical angle, the chest expanded, the muscles of waist, thigh and knees are stretched and taut. The spine is well articulated. Any one with cervical spondilitis should practise this cautiously, but when it can be accomplished with ease, the cervical vertebrae will benefit enormously and there will be an almost immediate reduction of any pain and tension in neck and shoulders.

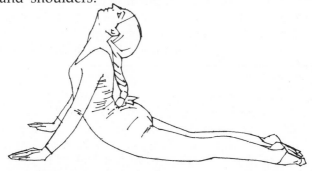

Figure 18 Bhujangāsana (Cobra Posture)

BHUJANGASANA (The Cobra) (Figure 18)
Technique:
Lie down, face prone, completely relaxed. Put the palms

on the floor exactly under the shoulders. The forehead rests on the mat. The legs are stretched out and kept close together. Breathe in and press the head back. Continuing to breathe in, begin to lift the upper torso, straightening the arms gradually and pressing back from the waist so that the whole body from the navel upward is pressed back in an arc. The pressure on the vertebrae of the neck gradually spreads lower and lower down the spine till it reaches the sacroiliac joints. From the waist down the body stays pressed firmly to the floor. The legs are together and the feet flat, not raised up on the toes. Exhale and begin to breathe slowly, if the pose is maintained for more than ten seconds. Exhale as the body is returned slowly to the mat, first relaxing the muscles from below and then gradually relaxing them, one by one, the lumbar, thoracic and cervical areas, until the spine is once again straight and the forehead rests on the mat. Gradually the time should be extended, till the pose can be held for thirty seconds. Till that time, repeat the pose three or four times for maximum benefit. When the pose can be held for thirty seconds, turn the head slowly over your shoulder to look back at the feet, first right and then left. This relieves tensions in the neck and shoulder area.

Bhujangi Mudra is to raise up in the Cobra pose but reverse the breath cycle and instead of inhaling, hiss out the breath like an angry cobra. Inhale as you lie on your mat, lift head and hiss as you raise the body up, pressing back from the waist. Hold position for some time, breathe in, exhale and return to starting position. This is excellent for neurasthenia, nerves or a depressed mood. It elevates the mood and acts as a tranquillizer, if repeated several times in succession.

Benefits:

Tension is loosened up in the entire spinal area right from the area behind the ears down to lower back. It is not at all a difficult posture and anyone with spinal pain, or cervical problems, should learn this asana first. It loosens up the spine, promotes circulation and stretches the abdomen, particularly the rectii. By alternate contraction and relaxation it adjusts minor displacements of the vertebra and makes the spine elastic. There is great relief from flatulence and dyspepsia and constipation is removed. It favourably influences menstrual complaints and other diseases of the female sexual organs. Back pain is almost immediately relieved if the posture is repeated several times with deep breathing. The back muscles are strengthened and regenerated. Every vertebra, ligament and tendon is tensed and relaxed alternately. The kidneys too are regenerated since during this asana blood is squeezed out of them and flows back vigorously, washing out impurities. The thyroid glands are stimulated and made to work efficiently. Those with over-active thyroids should not press the head back but keep it straight.

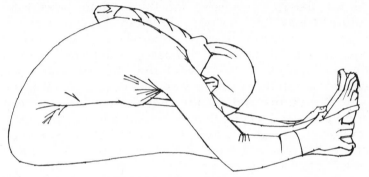

Figure 19 Paschimottanāsana (Trunk Bending Posture)

PASCHIMOTTANASANA (Trunk-Bending Posture) (Figure 19)
Technique:
Sit on your yoga mat with legs extended straight out in front. Exhale and bend forward to catch the ankles or feet with the hands. The knees remain completely stiff, elbows are lowered to the floor on either side of the knees. The position is held for some time and then a deep breath is inhaled while the body is straightened again, by first releasing the hold on toes or ankles, then lifting the head and finally relaxing the whole body. For people with stiff spines this is one of the most difficult of all asanas. I have met people in their twenties who find it impossible to bend much further than enables them to hold their shins and whose spines are so rigid that the head does not come anywhere near the knees. Be patient. Even the most rigid and inflexible of spines will gradually become supple with a daily yoga routine. Just bend as far as you can. Catching knees, shins or ankles — whichever is convenient. Keep the knees stiff at all times. Every day try and get your head

a little closer to your knees. Repeat the whole thing several times. When you can accomplish the perfect pose as in illustration, then hold the pose for thirty seconds or more, repeating only once. A variation, and a very useful one, is to begin this asana from a back-prone position, arms lying on the mat above the head. Breathe in, exhale and come up slowly as you exhale, to a sitting position and then bend forward over the knees to finish the pose. Repeat three or four times.

Benefits:

All the abdominal muscles and the rectii are powerfully contracted by this posture. The stomach, liver, spleen, kidneys and intestines work smoothly and it is a specific cure for constipation. If the asana is repeated several times, deposits of fat around the hips and abdomen disappear and the sexual organs, the rectum as well as the prostate, uterus and bladder are flushed with a fresh supply of blood so that their condition is toned and vastly improved. The thighs and the hamstrings are stretched and pulled, making them pliable and supple. When it is possible to hold the ankles or toes and put the head on the knees, then a further attempt should be made to bend only from the hips so that the back is lengthened and flattened and the head lies beyond the knees. The toes should be caught with the thumb and forefinger which can form hooks for this purpose. Diabetics should practise this pose regularly as it activates the pancreas which begins to produce insulin in the normal way.

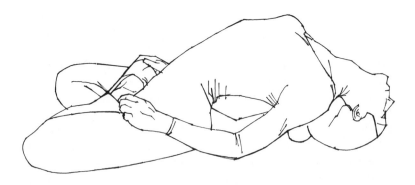

Figure 20 Matsyāsana (Fish Posture)

MATSYASANA (The Fish) (Figure 20)
See Figure 4 for Technique
Benefits:
In addition to being an excellent posture for mid-chest breathing Matsyasana has many other benefits. It is complementary to the Shoulder Stand and should be practised after it. The neck which was compressed in the shoulder stand is now bent back at a radical angle, draining the venous blood from the face, head and brain. The brain, the pituitary and pineal glands are supplied with oxygenated blood which forces them to work better. The neck is stretched, the muscles of the back contracted and the abdominal muscles tensed and pulled. The backward pressure of the head, with a fresh supply of blood forced into this area, activates the thyroid, and increases metabolism. After you have held the pose with deep, mid-chest breathing for as long as is comfortable, relax the arch of the back, flatten the head so that it lies in a normal position and, still keeping the legs in the lotus pose, fold the arms under the head. Continue to lie in this modified Fish Posture with deep breathing. This is particularly good for women as the sex organs are tightened and stretched and the muscular tone of the lower abdomen and pelvic organs are maintained. Kegel, Rout, McKenzie and others recommend the deliberate contracting and relaxing of the sphincter muscles to prevent incontinence and to tone up sexual organs. Matsyasana does this excellently, and as an added contribution to youthfulness the gluteal muscles and the rectum may be relaxed and contracted rhythmically so that they are made elastic and strong.

Special mudras for reconditioning the sex centres
While all the asanas contribute toward greater resilience, flexibility, health and stability of both the body and the mind, yoga has certain Mudras which are designed to tone up the sex organs either for greater virility or for sublimation. A healthy and normal sex life is not possible when there is congestion and tension in the pelvic area. Many of the poses which increase sexual virility and tone are used by the Yogis to control sexual desires and are often known as Brahmacharya Mudras or the Celibate Pose.

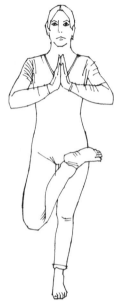

Figure 21 Vrikshāsana (Tree Posture)

VRIKSHASANA (Tree Posture) (Figure 21)
Technique:
Balance yourself firmly on one leg. Bend the knee of the other foot and place the foot on the thigh in a half-lotus position. You may need to use your hands to draw the foot into position. Fold the hands together at the chest and stand firmly without teetering or swaying for as long as possible, breathing deep and slow meanwhile. Choose a fixation point for your eyes about six feet away. Repeat with other leg.
Benefits:
This asana is to restore balance and equilibrium to the body by coordinating the mind with the appropriate brain centre. When balance is perfected then the sex centre, situated in the lower spine, is affected, improving sexual performance or relieving frustration and making celibacy possible. The lifted leg makes the pelvis supple, uncongested and tones up the entire region in this area.

VATSYAYUASANA (Colt-Face Posture) (Figure 22)
Technique:
This pose, where the angle of the legs is supposed to look

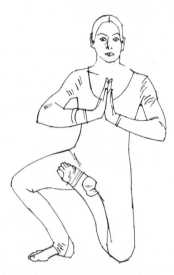

Figure 22 Vatsyayuāsana

like a horse's face, is done from Figure 21, the Tree
Posture. First balance on one leg and lift the other up into
the half-lotus. Steady the balance for a brief period and
then bend slowly and place the locked-up knee which is in
the half-lotus onto the floor, keeping the foot still firmly
against the thigh of the opposite leg. The other leg is
turned out for balance and the foot placed firmly, pointed
out. The hands are folded at the chest. In the beginning,
attain to this position by using your hands on either side,
placed on the floor for balance. Adjust the position of the
feet carefully. Hold briefly with deep, slow breathing,
straighten the bent knee and sit on the floor. Always
repeat each movement on the other side to produce equal
effects.

Benefits:

The exercise is aimed at making the pelvic area loose and
providing it with better circulation. The hips, the pelvic
area and the groin are generally not sufficiently exercised,
leading to congestion and tension in this area. Dr Swami
Gitananda says, 'A congested pelvis may be the cause of
abnormal sexual preoccupation. A healthy pelvis is the
first prerequisite of a healthy, normal sex life.' Energy is
not only restored but conserved instead of being dissipated.

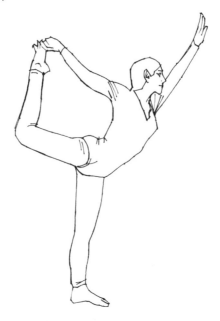

Figure 23 Natrajāsana (Pose of the Dancing Shiva)

NATRAJASANA (The Pose of the Dancing Shiva) (Figure 23)
Technique:
Stand firmly on your yoga mat. Bend the right knee and
lift it backwards. Take the right hand back and hold the
foot with the thumb and fingers, pulling the foot up as
high as possible. Stretch out the other hand in front of the
body, lean forwards slightly and balance on the left leg,
which is straight, knee pulled up tight and immobile. The
body tilts slightly forward to maintain the balance. A
fixation point for the eyes is found some six feet away on
the same level as the eyes. Hold the position without
swaying or teetering, breathing deeply meanwhile, for as
long as is possible. If you overbalance, regain your starting
position and begin again. If you still find this difficult then
hold on to a support with the free hand, till you learn to
balance correctly.
Benefit:
This is a very beautiful pose, dedicated to Shiva, Lord of
the Dance. It is a difficult balancing pose and develops
poise and a graceful figure. The legs, the knees, the
thighs, the shoulders and the chest are all toned and
strengthened. The pelvis area is made supple and the hips

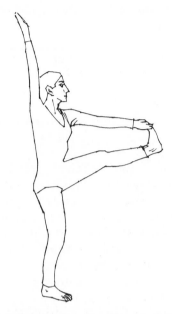

Figure 24 Hasta Padangusthāsana (Hand to Toe Posture)

exercised. It promotes and prolongs youth and retards the onset of old age. All the joints become very supple and the stomach and hips become slim and shapely. The pose should be practised on the other leg and both legs repeated twice for the greatest benefit. Anyone who practises this pose every day will never suffer from calcification of the bones. The urogenital and sexual glands are nourished and stimulated.

HASTAPADANGUSTASANA (Hand to Toe Posture) (Figure 24)
Technique:
Stand firmly on the mat with both legs together, hands at sides and back straight. Exhale and slowly, while exhaling, lift one leg straight forward till it is at right angles to the body. Do not bend the legs but keep both knees as straight as possible. Inhale and lift one arm straight into the air over the head, palm forward, while the other arm, the one on the same side as the lifted leg, is stretched out to catch the toe of the lifted leg. Retain this position for as long as possible with deep breathing. The head should be well poised on the neck and not bent forward or

backward. Exhale and return to starting position. Repeat with other leg.

In the beginning it might help to rest the lifted foot on a support which is high enough to keep the leg at right angles. In this way the hips become more limber, balance is perfected, and finally the pose may be accomplished without the help of the support. A further variation is to lift the legs sideways and then backwards, repeating each movement twice.

Benefits:

The hip flexion followed by deep breathing increases abdominal compression. The slow, alternate movements massage the abdominal viscera and the muscles of the lower abdomen, and at the same time the hips and the pelvis are exercised. Constipation and tension in these areas are removed and the waist and hips are kept slim and supple. This simple posture provides sufficient exercise for the deeper sex organs, aiding in the venous flow to these areas and supplying a much needed internal massage to the sex organs, especially of women.

UDDIYANA BANDHA (not illustrated)

Technique:

Neither Uddiyana Bandha nor the Nauli which follows it are, strictly speaking, asanas. Uddiyana is a Bandha or restraint and means 'upward flight'. When carried out properly it is quite spectacular and it also has spectacular results. It can be performed fairly easily by most people who do not have a lot of fat on their stomachs.

Nauli, on the other hand, is extremely difficult and may take several weeks, or even months, to learn. Stand on your yoga mat with feet about ten inches (25.5 cms) apart. Bend the knees slightly and bend forward, placing hands on top of thighs. The back is rounded. Inhale as in the complete yogic breath and then exhale completely. Now, with the breath still held out, suck in the abdomen, raise the diaphragm and expand the chest. The abdominal wall is now flattened against the spine and a hollow cavity is formed. The old yoga text, the Gheranda Samhita (III, 56) describes it thus: 'Stretching and pressing the abdomen to the back, and giving it the shape of a pond results in *Uddiyana Bandha*, which dispels old age and death.' While in this position, the anus and pelvic muscles are strongly contracted. When you can no longer hold the breath out, relax the muscles, allow the air to enter the lungs in a long, slow inhalation, and straighten up to starting position. Breath normally and then repeat the whole procedure once more. When you have learnt how to do this you can proceed to the next step which is called Agnisara Dhauti, the fanning of the Gastric fires.

AGNISARA DHAUTI (not illustrated)
Technique:
Having contracted the stomach after exhaling, now flap it in and out by allowing the muscles to relax and then pulling them against the spine in quick succession. The breath is still out and during the whole process no air must be allowed to enter the lungs.
Benefits:
No yoga practice can be deemed complete unless the stomach retraction is learned. Five minutes per day is all that is needed to achieve a flat belly, an end to constipation and stimulation of the adrenal and sex glands. The abdominal muscles are given a deep massage and lung tissue becomes elastic and therefore capable of withstanding infection. The large intestine and the diaphragm are lifted, and compressed, and peristaltic activity encouraged. The viscera are kneaded and massaged, and circulation in this area speeded up. In fact the whole of the digestive tract is activated and the liver, just beneath the diaphragm, is decongested while the pancreas is stimulated. With the hollowing out of the thoracic cage the lungs and heart get a beneficial massage. I have found that many Western students have absolutely rigid and motionless diaphragms and they have absolutely no idea how to breathe in this area. This exercise restores mobility to the diaphragm and makes yogic breathing much easier. Sexual organs and glands in both males and females are revived and rejuvenated. The ovaries and testes are maintained in good condition. The urinary system is also encouraged to function properly. Since the spine and the sympathetic nerves adjoining it get a rich supply of blood the whole nervous system begins to work harmoniously for good health.

NAULI (not illustrated)
Technique:
Stand as for Uddiyana Bandha. Exhale and suck in the abdominal wall. Keeping the stomach muscles totally retracted, try and isolate the abdominal recti in the centre so that they stand in a prominent ridge. Contract the hips muscles so that pressure is exerted just above the pubic bones. You will not be able to do this in the beginning but make the attempt. When this is successful and the central muscles are isolated, then try and roll them to the left and right. The muscle on the right is relaxed while the left muscle is rolled to the left. The muscle on the left is then relaxed while the right muscle is rolled to the right. An adept practitioner does this so smoothly that it looks as if one muscle is being rotated from left to right and back again. Getting someone to help you learn this is advisable. Meanwhile you can start to practise Uddiyana and the Agnisara Dhauti which will have spectacular results.
Benefits:
The benefits of Nauli are much the same as Uddiyana, only more so. The rolling of the recti muscles in both directions stretches the intestines and massages them as no other exercise can do. The bowels will function normally and constipation can never occur if this is practised.

Since both these yogic practices have such powerful benefits there are also certain safeguards and limitations to follow. The bladder and bowel must be emptied before they are performed. The stomach should also be empty and no food should have been taken for at least four hours previously. Children should not be allowed to practice this until fourteen years of age. Koestler, when he first saw this yogic exercise, was both fascinated and horrified. He wrote: 'The Yogi began by drawing in the abdominal muscles while forcing the viscera and diaphragm upward until a large hollow cavity appeared under the ribs, a kind of incredible grotto in the flesh, and the *obliqui abdomini*, the two transversal muscles stuck out in a rather horrifying manner as on anatomical figures stripped of skin.'

Yes, it is very impressive, very effective and takes no more than five minutes a day. Every one should practise Uddiyana Bandha and the 'fanning of gastric fires' that follows, even if they never achieve Nauli. Relax after this fairly strenous workout, with some deep rhythmical breathing.

Another excellent exercise for the sex muscles is Mula-Bandha and its corollary, Ashwini Mudra. These tone up the bladder, the rectum and the sex muscles. They recondition the ovaries and testes, and prevent complications, minor growths and erosion of the cervix, and of the vas deferens and the prostate in men. They are easy to perform and should be done every single day, without fail.

MULA-BANDHA (Contraction of the Anal and Pelvic Muṣcles)
(not illustrated)
Mula means 'root' and Bandha means 'contraction' or 'seal'! In this posture the sex organs, the rectum and the pelvic organs are exercised and contracted.
Technique:
This posture may be done standing, sitting or lying. Inhale deeply and then exhale. With the breath held out contract the ring of muscles around the anus tightly, causing the whole pelvic region to contract. Hold tight for a few moments and then relax and repeat the exercise ten times, exhaling before tightening the muscles and inhaling when they are relaxed. Women should also contract the sphincter muscles at the same time. Imagine that you are holding a coin between your buttocks and are holding tight to prevent it dropping. This will contract the muscles of the pelvic floor. If the sphincter muscles are tightly contracted, the muscles which affect urination are controlled. Do both simultaneously ten times, repeating the whole thing at least three times a day.

ASHWINI MUDRA (not illustrated)
This is very similar to the above exercise except that the breath is not exhaled and kept out. Breathing is normal while the muscles of the rectum are contracted and relaxed rapidly, about ten times at one stretch. Relax and repeat again, several times.
Benefits:
Both these exercises should be practised by everyone, male or female, at least three times a day. They are very easy to perform, take little time and can be done anywhere. These muscles, if not properly exercised, get

slack and loose with age or with child-bearing. They tend to atrophy and waste away, impairing the elasticity of the tissue. The bladder will then prolapse and the muscles of the anus, the pelvic muscles and the sexual muscles all lose tone. Regular practice will keep the genital and sexual organs healthy, and the prostate gland and gonads in good condition. The effects of these exercises will be felt only after a few weeks so remember to practise every single day. The Yogis say excessive sexual desires are also controlled and energy is not dissipated. The sexual glands are regenerated and made healthy, for healthy sex or for sublimation.

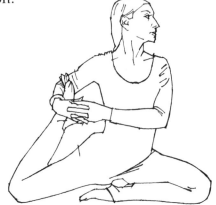

Figure 25 Vamadevāsana (The Pose of Shiva)

VAMADEVASANA (The Pose of Shiva) (Figure 25)
Technique:
Kneel on your yoga mat. Stretch the right leg out straight behind and tuck the left foot into the groin, toes pointing back, knee flat on floor. Keep the torso stretched up. Now bend the extended leg and catch the foot with both hands bound together, so that it is caught between the hands. The body faces toward the front, the head looking directly over the left shoulder. An extension of this admittedly difficult but very beautiful pose, is to draw up the bent foot and lock it under the rib cage. This is one of the *karanas* or movements of the dancing Shiva. The breathing is normal, slow and deep. Hold the position for a few moments and then relax and repeat on the other side. In the beginning it is enough to sit with the leg extended at the back and the other foot tucked into the groin. Get the feel of this position. You may need to support yourself

with your hands on the floor, on either side of the front knee. Take it slow and easy. There is no hurry and the benefits are enormous.

Benefits:

One look at the illustration will show you the marvellous stretch of pelvis, hips, thighs and the urogenital area. Stiffness of the legs and knees are cured, the genital organs are kept healthy by fresh blood circulating in this area, the waist is made slim and supple, and sexual energy is restored.

Asanas for arthritis, diabetes and other problems

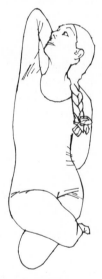

Figure 26 Gomukhāsana (Cow-Face Posture)

GOMUKHASANA (The Cow-Face Posture) (Figure 26)
Technique:

Kneel on your yoga mat. Sit back on one heel so that the rectum fits precisely over the heel. Cross the other leg over the thigh, pressing the foot tightly back. Take one arm over the shoulder, with the palm down on the back. Take other arm up from below and clasp fingers of both hands behind back. The elbow of the arm over the shoulder is kept straight and high. Turn the head and look up at the lifted elbow. Pull up with the lifted arm and down with the other so that the shoulders are pulled and stretched.

Do not allow the torso to twist off to one side. Breath deeply and keep the stomach well pulled in. The benefits of this pose are increased if the muscles around the anus and the pelvis are rhythmically contracted and relaxed. Repeat after holding the pose for as long as possible, on both sides.

Benefits:

The muscles of the neck, the shoulders, the back and the vertebral column are pulled and exercised. Those suffering from stiff necks and cervical spondylosis will benefit, as well as those with bursitis of the shoulders. Arthritic deposits in knees, hips and ankles are dissolved and the muscles of the abdominal wall and pelvis are exercised and get a good supply of fresh blood. Most people are unable to grasp the hands at the back, in which case a handkerchief or scarf should be used to bridge the gap. The hands can gradually be moved closer and closer till they can eventually be locked together. Inability to lock the hands behind the back on both sides means unequal development of muscles or extreme stiffness.

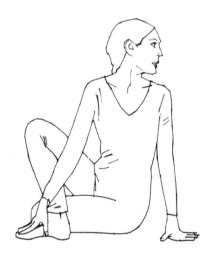

Figure 27 Marichyāsana (Spinal Twist)

MARICHYASANA (The Spinal Twist) (Figure 27)
Technique:
Sit on the yoga mat with the legs extended straight out in

front. Bend the left leg at the knee and place the left foot near the right hip. Bend the right knee and cross over the bent left leg so that the foot lies alongside the left knee. With the right hand catch hold of the right foot. Exhale and turn the body slowly to look over the left shoulder. The left hand is placed down on the floor for support. Breathe in and out smoothly while holding the pose for thirty seconds. Relax, and repeat on other side.

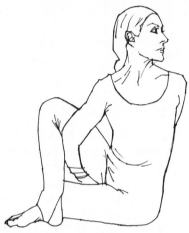

Figure 28 Marichyāsana (Variation I)

MARICHYASANA (Variation 1) (Figure 28)
Instead of holding the right foot with the right hand, lock the arms behind the back from under the thigh. The body is twisted to the left as far as possible, the head looking over the left shoulder with some tension. Breathe deeply in and out and hold the position for thirty seconds. Relax and repeat on other side.

MARICHYASANA (Variation 2) (Figure 29)
In this pose, the arms are locked behind the back over the knee. The torso is twisted off to the left. Breathe in and out and hold the position for thirty seconds. Relax and repeat on other side.
Benefits:
If each pose is held for thirty seconds it will take three minutes to complete the three variations. The abdominal muscles are well exercised and stiffness in shoulders, arms, knees and ankles removed. The radical turning of

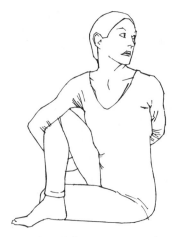

Figure 29 Marichyāsana (Variation II)

the head, with some tension, loosens up this area. The waist, which is twisted in both directions, becomes slimmer and the locked arms create a pull which is excellent for upper arm flab. Because of the pull and stretch of the muscles and joints, circulation is improved and the synovial fluid restored. This removes stiffness and pain, strengthens bones and increases flexibility, all normal conditions of advancing age.

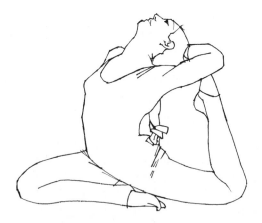

Figure 30 Rajkapotāsana (The Royal Pigeon)

RAJKAPOTASANA (The Royal Pigeon) (Figure 30)
Technique:
Kneel on your yoga mat. Sit down with the right knee bent

and the right foot placed so that the heel touches the groin. Stretch the other leg back. Take a deep breath and exhale. Bend the foot of the left leg up, and catch the foot with the locked arms. The torso is bent backward and head rests on the locked arms. The head is tilted back, looking up at the sky. An advanced position is to bend the body and head even further back so that the sole of the foot touches the forehead. The chest is pushed well forward (like a pigeon). In the beginning it is enough to simply bend the foot and place it against the groin while the other is extended back. Place both hands on either side of the knee on the floor and bend and arch the back and head as far as possible. This is a very beautiful but extremely difficult posture. Those who are young and supple might be able to do it but for those over forty it will prove difficult. Nevertheless, it is well worth attempting even if the complete pose is not achieved. Inhale and relax. Repeat on both sides twice.

Benefits:
This pose will prevent calcification of the bones and make the whole body very limber and supple. Knees, ankles, elbows, neck, shoulders, arms, hips, thighs, and back are all stretched and tensed, increasing circulation and pouring a fresh supply of rejuvenating blood through the veins. The pubic region too gets a fresh supply of blood and the thyroids, parathyroids, adrenals and gonads are stimulated, increasing vitality. Even a modified version will produce excellent benefits. One symptom of old age is the disinclination to try anything new or difficult. Attempting something new is in itself a challenge, and an incentive to think young.

HALASANA (The Plough Posture) (Figure 31)
Technique:
Lie down on the floor in a back supine position with the arms at the sides, and the feet together. Breathe in and lift both legs together to a perpendicular position. Breathe out and continue to carry the legs over the head till they touch the floor at the back. Lock the hands together and breathe so that the breath comes slow and deep. The legs should be kept together and straight, the knees stiff. The arms are flat on the floor, hands locked together. The posture may be maintained for as long as it is comfortable before

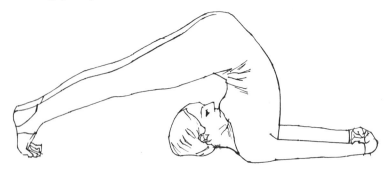

Figure 31 Halāsana (Plough Posture)

returning slowly to the floor, rolling the body down from shoulders, down the mid-back and finally the lower back till you are once again lying with the back supine on the floor. The head must be kept firmly on the mat while returning to the starting position.

In the beginning, those who have very stiff spines will not be able to touch their feet down beyond the head. Put a pile of cushions behind you and bring the feet down on this support. Gradually remove one cushion at a time till the feet rest on the floor. Even when this happens you will find that the feet are very close to the head. Concentrate every day on pushing the feet just a little further till the chin is pressed up against the chest and the hips are directly over the head.

Start with only one movement a day, gradually working up to three rounds and holding the position a little longer each day. Variations are to bring the hands up and fold them under the head or to stretch the arms out behind the head and catch the toes. A Kriya or movement is to separate the legs widely and bring them together again, two or three times while still in the same position. Another variation is to bend the knees and place them on either side of the head.

Benefits:

While most yoga postures stretch the spine, either forward, backward or sideways, this position stretches the spine to the point where the vertebrae are pulled as though in traction, releasing them from pressure and relieving the strain which occurs while in the upright position. Because of the stretch, circulation speeds up and there is a steady improvement in the tone and activity of the spine, increasing its pliancy and mobility. Because of the inverted intra-abdominal pressure, there is proper drainage and functioning of the viscera and the pelvic organs are replaced in their correct position. The ligaments and supporting muscles of the sexual organs are strengthened, the nerves purified and the mind made calm and tranquil. The neck too is stretched, the legs, ankles, thighs and hips are all tensed and relaxed in a very beneficial manner. The thyroid glands, compressed during the stationary part of the pose, are activated and their functions regularized. This pose has a very great effect on the youthfulness of the body, as hormones are secreted which aid the smoothness and fresh appearance of the skin. Halasana has a reviving effect on tired and exhausted bodies. It acts like a tonic and should be tried by anyone who feels stiff and fatigued after a long day at the office. Just two or three minutes in this pose, or alternately, the repetition of the posture two or three times, is sufficient to unwind stiff, aching muscles, and leave the body feeling relaxed and energized.

The spleen, the sexual glands, and the pancreas are all massaged and toned and diabetics should practise this asana every day, beginning easily. Because of the compression of the abdominal organs, constipation is relieved. People who suffer from low blood pressure, slow metabolism, and physical or mental laziness should practise Halasana three times a day. They will soon see a difference. Bodies which are fat, bulgy and out of proportion will be reshaped with the practice of Halasana.

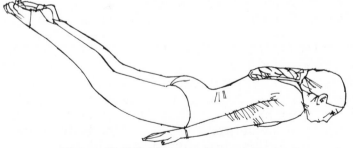

Figure 32 Salabhāsana (Locust Posture)

SALBHASANA (Locust Posture) (Figure 32)
Technique:
Lie face down on your yoga mat. The head is stretched so

that the chin rests on the floor, the arms lie alongside the body, palms flat down. The feet are together, the legs stretched out straight. Inhale deeply and lift both legs into the air as high as possible. Hold position for as long as possible, exhale and lower the feet and legs. Repeat this two or three times. In the beginning you may clench the hands into fists and push them under the thighs to help in the lifting of the legs. You may lift only an inch (2.5 cms) or so at first, but do not give up. Continue practising every single day. The Ardha-Salbhasana is to lift one leg at a time on the inhaled breath. Inhale, lift one leg, hold the position, exhale and lower the leg. Repeat with the other leg, at least twice on either side.

Benefits:

This is one of the best exercises for lower back pain and has been adopted by many orthopaedic surgeons who are treating lower disc problems or sciatica of the lower back muscles. Intra-abdominal pressure is increased and the pelvis and legs are strengthened. Because the stomach is pressed against the floor while the legs are lifted, the abdominal organs are subjected to a powerful massage and constipation is cured. A large supply of blood forces the intestines to work properly. The alternate tensing and relaxing of the muscles affects the digestive glands. Anyone who suffers from lower back pain, (and that must include around fifty per cent of all people) should practise this posture with both one leg at a time and then with both legs together. If it is impossible to get the legs up more than an inch (2.5 cms) or so, get someone to stand behind and gently lift the legs, drawing them up as far as possible. The relief from back pain will be startling.

DHANURASANA (The Bow) (Figure 33)

Technique:

Lie face down on your yoga mat, with the feet together and legs stretched out, your forehead on mat. Inhale slowly, grasp the ankles with the hands (note the position of hands in the illustration) and pull the body up into a bow. The head should be forced back with some tension and the arms tugged so that the shoulders are well stretched. The feet should be raised so that they are higher than the head. Hold position for as long as is comfortable and then exhale and relax.

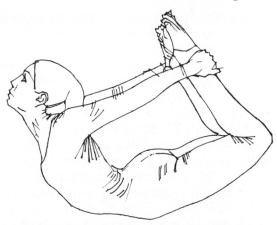

Figure 33 Dhanurāsana (Bow Posture)

Many of my students find it impossible, in the initial stages, to lift their knees even half an inch (a centimetre) from the floor. They tug the ankles, lift their heads and seem stuck to the floor. They are in despair since the bow seems a fairly simple posture. I can only assure you, as I do them, that as the spine becomes more pliable, and all the joints of the body more flexible, the knees will lift off the floor, at first only fractionally perhaps, but with constant practice you can achieve this beautiful pose. Just feel that whatever stretch you have achieved is doing you good, making you more flexible, bringing fresh blood to the spine.

From this static position you can do *Dhanush Kriya*. Rock forwards on to the chest on an exhaled breath, so that the feet come high over the head, rock back on to the abdominal region, still with the breath held out. Rock back and forth, rest, and repeat the whole sequence once more. The breath is exhaled in order to protect the internal organs as the body is rocked back and forth.
Benefits:
Degeneration of the spine, rigidity, stiffness, and aches and pains in the back are all cured by this asana. The abdominal area is given a deep and thorough massage (especially if you rock back and forth) and layers of fat on the belly disappear. The waist, and hips become slim and supple and the muscle of the legs, knees, and thighs are stretched and exercised strongly, eliminating rheumatism pains. All kinds of bowel congestion is removed and

peristaltic activity speeds up, improving digestion and removing constipation. Premature calcification of the bones can never occur in those who diligently practise Dhanurasana every day. Bursitis of the shoulders and cervical spondilitis are cured and almost immediate relief is experienced when there is excruciating pain. Children can do this very easily and women seem better at it than men. Everyone should practise it, however. Remember to keep the feet together when the legs are lifted. The knees too should be together and not spread apart because when the pull is felt the knees and the shoulders should be aligned so that there is no unequal stretching of the thigh muscles. According to Dr Rele, if the knees are kept apart 'it puts a greater strain on the muscles which lie on the outer side of the thighs and more particularly on the Tensor Fascia Lata. The strain is manifested by a tearing pain on the outer and lower border of the patella to which it is attached.' When the knees are kept together there is no danger of this.

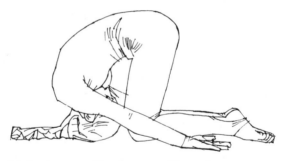

Figure 34 Paripurna Shashāsana (Completed Hare Posture)

PARIPURNA SHASHASANA (Completed Hare Posture) (Figure 34)
Technique:
Sit on your yoga mat in *Vajrasana* (Figure 4) and bend forward into Dharmikasana (Figure 8). Breathe in and roll up on to the head, lifting right off the heels. The arms lie alongside the legs, the thighs from the knee right up to the hip are straight and at right angles to the lower legs. The neck is turned under to provide an even greater curve to the top of the spine. Breathe out and return to Dharmikasana. Inhale and sit up in Vajrasana. The entire sequence should be repeated at least thrice.

Benefits:
This posture, continuing on from Vajrasana and Dharmi-kasana, is not at all difficult and can be done by almost everyone. If the straight knee-to-hip posture cannot be done at first, just bend over as far as is possible. It has benefits out of all proportion to the effort necessary to attain it. The thyroid-para-thyroid gland complex is stimulated, the windpipe is stretched and natural elasticity is returned to the bronchial tubes. The spine has seven cervical bones, twelve dorsal or thoracic bones in the high and middle back, five lumbar or lower back bones, five bones fused together in the sacrum and five more in the coccygeal or tail-bone area. Twenty-five of these bones need to remain articulated or movement and flexibility of the spine is severely restricted. This asana pulls and stretches all the vertebrae to the point where the cerebro-spinal fluids cushioning the spinal cord and the brain are relieved of excess pressure. In this posture the spine shows an increase in length of twenty to twenty-five per cent above the straight sitting position. This in itself is tension-relieving. It should be practised regularly by anyone with cervical pain or neck tension and also by those with very rigid and inflexible spines. As a preliminary to more difficult positions it is excellent for loosening up the spine and making it more flexible.

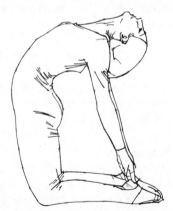

Figure 35 Ushtrāsana (Camel Posture)

USHTHRASANA (The Camel) (Figure 35)
Technique:
Sit on the heels in Vajrasana (Figure 5). Exhale. Inhale and

lift the buttocks off the heels. Bend the back till the heels can be caught with the hands. Push the lower part of the body, the legs and abdominal area, forwards, arch the body and drop the head between the shoulders. Breathe out forcefully and breathe in again. Do this several times. The breath will be concentrated in the lower abdominal lobes of the lungs. Lift off the hands and straighten the body as you inhale. Exhale and sit back on heels. Do this only once in the beginning, and after a week or two's practice do it three times.

Benefits:

Full spinal articulation is achieved, relieving stiffness, aches and pains. The neck is made supple and tension in this area relieved. The lungs benefit from the deep, controlled breathing, enlarging, expanding and rejuvenating the various nerves affected by the pressures. People with drooping backs, hunched shoulders, or dowager's humps should practise this regularly every day. Elderly people can also practise this pose with great advantage. Instead of holding the heels they can simply lean back, and dangle the arms loosely at the sides, dropping the head and neck back as far as possible. If there is any danger of falling over, a friend can help by putting a restraining hand on the mid-back to prevent losing balance. Abdominal organs are toned and the chest, which is fully expanded in this posture, becomes broad and well-developed.

SANTULASANA (Stretching Pose) (Figure 36)
Technique:

Stand up straight on your yoga mat, hands at the sides, feet together. The eyes should be looking straight ahead. Balance on the left leg and fold the right one back at the knee, bringing the heel up against the hip. Lock both hands around the foot and press it as close as possible to the hip. The body will lean slightly forward, the head should be turned to look over the left shoulder. Balance as long as possible in this graceful position, breathing deep and slow. Release the hand-lock, drop the foot back to the mat and relax. Repeat with the other leg. Do this twice on either side.

Benefits:

Not only does this improve balance and grace but it makes

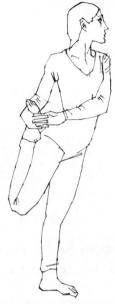

Figure 36 Santulāsana (Stretching Posture)

all the joints, especially of the legs, very flexible. Stiffness and rigidity are removed and pains in the knees, ankles and heels are reduced. Many old people, whether through overweight or through stiffness, have stiff and painful knees and they walk with a rolling, listing motion, to ease pressure on their knees. Often the knees become enlarged and swollen. Practise of this posture will bring great mobility to the leg joints. If there is danger of tipping over, hold on with one hand to the back of a chair or some other support, and pull the heel close to the hip with the other hand.

UTTANAPADASANA (Leg-Lifting Posture) (Figure 37)
Technique:
Lie down on the back on your yoga mat with the feet together and the hands comfortably at sides. The head is neither tilted back nor forward. Start rhythmic breathing to the count of 8x4x8x4. Now lift the legs, both together to the count of 8. Keep the knees straight. Hold the lift to a count of 4, then slowly exhale and count to 8. Hold the position with legs relaxed on the mat to the count of 4. Inhale — 8, hold — 4, exhale — 8, hold out — 4. Repeat

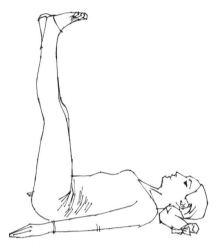

Figure 37 Uttanapada Asana (Leg-Lifting Posture)

the movements three to six times with the same slow, rhythmic breathing. Relax with rhythmic breathing. Variations on this double legs lift is to lift the legs together and when in the position in Figure 37, hold the breath and then exhale and lower the legs after opening them in a wide arc back to the floor. A further variation is to scissor the legs while lifting, hold them together in the high leg lift and scissor them back to the floor, using the inhaled and exhaled breaths for lifting and lowering the legs. If you find this too strenuous then try one leg at a time, using the same slow count of 8x4x8x4 and repeating the movement at least twice on each side.

Benefits:

Very strong abdominal muscles are built with these asanas. Strong back muscles (especially the lower back) are built as well if this asana is done first with one leg (to lessen the strain) and then with both legs together. The abdominal muscles are massaged both internally and externally by the movements, curing digestive disorders and constipation and removing fat from the stomach area. The hip joints are exercised mildly and become more flexible. The waist, buttocks and hips are all fed with a fresh supply of blood. Because abdominal strength is built up, hernias, prolapsed muscles and organs of the abdomen such as the uterus and rectum, are cured or prevented.

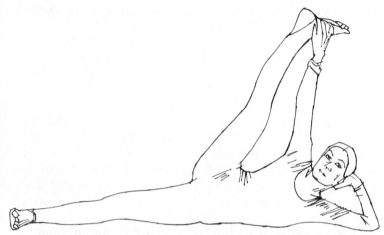

Figure 38 Anantāsana (Vishnu's Couch Posture)

ANANTASANA (Vishnu's Couch Posture) (Figure 38)
Technique:
Lie flat on the back on your yoga mat. Exhale and turn on the left side, lying straight with feet stretched out and together. Raise the head, bend the left arm at the elbow and support the head, just above the ear, on the hand. Breathe normally in this position for a few seconds. Inhale and bend the right knee and catch the toes with the right hand. Straighten the knee and pull the leg up vertically as high and as straight as you can. Exhale and breathe normally as you hold the position for fifteen seconds or longer. Your hip joints will have to adjust to this pose. Exhale, release the toe-hold, and return the leg to the mat. Lower the head and roll over on the back. Repeat the whole sequence on the other side. In yoga the right side is always first charged and balanced and then the left.
Benefits:
Flabby abdominal muscles will soon tone up and become hard. It is a 'firming position' and everything — legs, thighs, hips, abdomen and waist — are all exercised, stretched radically, pulled and relaxed again. If you pull the foot up closer to the head you will feel the wonderful stretch on the pelvic and hip muscles. Blood circulation speeds up and the whole abdominal area and the organs inside benefit. Cellulite on hips and thighs is dissolved and the arms are made slim and strong. The pelvic area and hamstring muscles are stretched and toned. Low

backaches are relieved and the development of hernias prevented.

It is a good idea to do all three of the leg-lifting asanas one after the other for greatest benefit. Begin with Figure 37, the double or single leg-lifts, while lying on your back. Turn over on the left and do Anantasana (Figure 38), turn over on your face and do Salbhasana (Figure 32), lifting your legs, singly or together from a face-prone position; then turn over on your right and repeat the side-lifing asana which you have just learnt. These postures, one after the other give you the most complete work-out that you could ever get, for the lower back, pelvic area, abdominal area and legs. They are powerful postures which will correct metabolic disorders and give the body a chance to work and adjust in a healthy, normal manner.

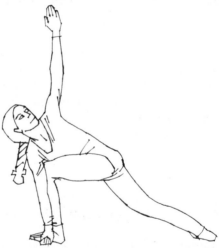

Figure 39 Parsvakonāsana (Perfected Angle Posture)

PARSVAKONASANA (Perfected, Angle Posture) (Figure 39)
Technique:
Parsva means side, and Kona is an angle. Stand on your yoga mat, feet together, arms at sides. Spread legs apart about 4 feet (1.22 metres) wide. Raise the arms sideways in line with the shoulders, palms down. Turn the right foot sideways 90° to the right and the left foot 60° to the right, keeping the left leg tightly stretched. Bend the right knee so that the thigh and calf form a right angle. Exhale and bring the right arm over the right knee. Close the hand into a fist and place it on the outer side of the right foot. Inhale,

give a twist to the spine and lift the left arm high into the air. Turn the head and look up at the palm of the outstretched hand. The knee of the outstretched leg should be kept stiff and unbending. Breathe slow and deep as you hold this tense position for ten to thirty seconds. Inhale, lift the right arm from its position on the floor, turn the neck and bring the head back to a straight position and lift the body up. With a jump, bring feet together. Relax. Repeat on other side, reversing the whole process.

Benefits:

This is a marvellous stretch for the entire body. You will feel the pull on shoulders, waist, abdomen, hips, thighs and legs. Fat is reduced around the waist and hips and sciatic and arthritic pains are greatly relieved. The abdominal organs are contracted, aiding elimination and digestion. The blood will circulate rapidly, rejuvenating all muscles and joints. The spine is made mobile and the neck relieved of tension. People who have very stiff joints should practise this asana every day. In the beginning it is enough simply to stand with feet wide apart and bend the knee of one leg. Lean the body slightly forward and stretch. When you get used to this and become a little more supple, add the torso twist with the two arms in their proper positions. This will take some time but the benefits in loosening up stiff muscles and joints is tremendous.

SHAVASANA (The Relaxation Posture) (not illustrated)
Technique:

Lie on your back stretched to full length in a quiet spot. Bring the heels together and then let the feet fall apart. The arms are relaxed along the sides of the body, palms up or down — whichever feels better. The head should be in a straight position, neither pressed down into the neck nor tilted back. Flatten the back so that it lies comfortably on the mat. Close the eyes. Begin by breathing deeply, the rhythmic 8x4x8x4 breath, to bring a sense of harmony to the body. Now imagine that your bones have all dissolved and your skin is stuffed with sawdust or rags, like a rag doll. Feel that the floor on which you are lying has magnetic properties, drawing your body down, down. Feel the heaviness as the body relaxes. Now turn your mind to the feet. Imagine your feet without tension, soft, relaxed. Take this feeling slowly up to the heels, ankles, calves, knees and thighs. Feel as though from the thighs down you are muscleless, jointless and floppy, like a doll. Now relax the buttocks and hips, the abdominal and pelvic areas, the lower back, mid-back, waist, chest and upper back, shoulders and neck. Imagine that from the neck down you are filled with sawdust. There are no muscles, joints or bones to tense up. Now take your attention down to the fingers. Relax them, then the palms, wrists, forearms, elbows, upper arms and back to the shoulders. Below the neck there is no tension anywhere. Now to the most difficult part: relaxing the face and head. Relax the lower jaw, open mouth slightly and part lips so that the teeth are not clenched. Relax the muscles of the cheeks, the eyes, the forehead and continue on to the top of the head and around the back of the head. Relax tension around the ears and return to the centre of the forehead, between the eyebrows, the third eye or *Ajna Chakra*. Breathe slowly, concentrating your attention on this spot. If you are really relaxed, the breathing will get slower and slower and almost stop as you go into a deep state of total relaxation. Stay in this pose for a minimum of ten minutes before sitting up slowly and coming back to life. It is absolutely imperative that when you are in this deep, deep state of total relaxation, nothing disturbs you. Lock yourself up so that no door bells, no telephone bells or any other distractions disturb you. It is dangerous to be woken suddenly from this state.

Benefits:

Shavasana is always done at the end of your yoga practice so that muscles which have been tensed, tugged, pulled, twisted and compressed, are allowed to relax. It is a valuable discipline to learn so that you can lie down (always on a hard, flat surface) when tense or tired and allow all tension to flow out of you. If you lie with the head to the north and feet to the south, you will be taking advantage of the 'magnetic polarity flow along the surface of the earth'. The posture not only relaxes and eases muscular tension but also it calms and soothes the mind, makes it easy to abstract oneself from all the daily worries and anxieties that beset any normal human being, and prepares the mind for meditation practice. One should attempt to consciously divest the mind of all though — trying to *still the mind* as in Zen and achieve a state of 'no mind'. Once this is learnt it is of the greatest benefit in everyday life. The mind, for the most part, is not thinking deep thoughts, but simply churning round and around in a state of distracted, inner dialogue that adds greatly to tension and nervousness. The Yogis say that one should think only when there is something to think about, for the rest, try and achieve the 'no mind', which helps to make the mind clear and alert instead of foggy and confused. Conscious relaxation, when mastered and practised regularly between intervals of work and physical effort, is one of the best assets for beauty, health, vigour and longevity. Shavasana should also be resorted to between different asanas, in order to allow the muscles to relax. Mini relaxation periods are of the greatest benefit during the practice of asanas and the old Yogic texts, recommend them very highly. Finish every yoga practice with this pose.

How to get the most out of yoga practice
It is preferable to practise in a room in which there will be no interruptions. If possible, lock your door and make the family understand that this is *your* time in which you are to be left alone. This will enable you to concentrate on what you are doing. Without perfect concentration the value of all yogic practices is considerably lessened. Pay special attention to the breath. When you breathe in, visualise prana flowing and energizing your entire body. When you breathe out, direct that prana to various parts of the body. Your room should be clean, airy and free fom cigarette fumes. Smoking, alcohol and excessive drinking of tea and coffee should not be indulged in. Start your practice with a few stretching exercises (see end of chapter) which release tension and direct the mind in the proper direction. Your attitude should be one of anticipation and acceptance for the good you will be doing both body and mind. Anxiety, fear, anger, worry, rage, envy and restlessness should not be allowed to enter your yoga room. Practice with caution. Do not attempt too much in the beginning. Follow the chart for week by week progress.

During menstruation women should not practise any

asanas except the sitting postures and the relaxation posture. Breathing should be continued without any retention of breath. This can prove very beneficial in releasing local tension and relieving cramps and pain. Certain asanas may be practised throughout the nine months of pregnancy. All of the sitting postures are very good as well as Baddhakonasana (Figure 8), Vrikshasana (Figure 21), Natrajasana (Figure 23) and Gomukhasana (Figure 26). All will make the hips and pelvis supple and keep the body in good condition.

If you feel exhausted, tired and uneasy after your practice then you are doing something wrong and you should get guidance from a competent teacher. You should feel light, energized, relaxed and ready for anything. If you have only a short time, don't hurry through the practice. Reduce the number of asanas, so that you can spend sufficient time on each. Doing a lot of asanas in a hurry and without proper concentration will do you little good. A few asanas, properly and correctly done, will yield great benefits.

When you have practised for some time regularly, you should begin to notice a difference in your body, mind and emotions. The body will be more supple, the weight will be more evenly distributed and bulges and layers of fat will have disappeared. Your energy level should be high and stamina and resistance will have improved to an unbelievable extent. Your mind should be more calm and peaceful and your emotions positive and outgoing. You will sleep better, eat better (of the correct foods), your digestion will be good and constipation will have been eliminated.

It is a good idea not only to fast one day each week, drinking only water with lemon juice and a little honey, but also to control speech, keeping silent for twenty-four hours and speaking only when it is absolutely necessary and you really have something to say. A lot of precious energy is dissipated in small, babbling talk, which comes flowing out like water from a tap, dissipating vital energy and muddling up the mind. Keep silent and store up positive energy and strengthen your health.

If you live in a high-rise building, try to get out once a week or more often to walk on the earth and keep in contact with the earth's healing and magnetic forces.

Psychologists have discovered that people who live in high-rise buildings suffer from anxiety, neuroses and many kinds of psychosomatic ailments. Walk on a beach, in a park, in a garden or country lane. If you can take your shoes off so much the better. Allow the sun and the wind and the magnetic forces of the earth to provide their healing and rejuvenating effects.

Learn to be moderate in everything. The Juan Mascaró version of the *Bhagvad Gita* says: 'Yoga is not for him who eats too much, or for him who eats too little; not for him who sleeps too much or for him who sleeps too little. Yoga is harmony. Harmony in eating and resting, in sleeping and keeping awake; a perfection in whatever one does. This is the Yoga that gives peace from all pain. When the mind of the Yogi is in harmony and finds rest in the Spirit within, all restless desires gone, then he is a Yukta, one in God. Then his soul is a lamp whose light is steady, for it burns in a shelter where no winds come.'

You will notice in the practice charts that asanas are generally grouped so that a forward-bending one is followed by a backward-bend and so on. It is not, however, absolutely necessary to be rigid about this. There are some yoga teachers who insist that exactly the same asanas should be practised every day, in exactly the same order. If you do this you are going to lose a lot of the fun and adventure involved in learning yoga. Not all bodies are the same and you might discover some asanas which make you feel so good that you will want to repeat them several times a day, like a Japanese pupil of mine with severe low back pain. She discovered that Vyaghrah Asana (The Tiger Pose) and Bhujangasana (the Cobra) made her feel so good she would do them several times a day, while something was simmering away on the stove. Moreover, if you restrict yourself to a certain basic set of asanas, you may never have the joy of trying out new and more difficult asanas, and finding that you can do them to perfection. Your body is now more supple, stronger, more resilient. It is *ready* to try out something new. Ready to feel the pull of new muscles and to get even more benefits from a Yoga session. Not for nothing did the ancient Rishis invent so many different asanas. My advice is to learn first the ones that come easily to you — and this is not always the same one for everyone. What is easy and simple for me could be very difficult indeed for you and vice versa. When the easy ones have been perfected, then go on to something more difficult and which appeals to you. This is very important. Sometimes you could develop an aversion to some particular asanas. Let them be: there are many others to choose from. Don't let anyone tell you that unless you can sit in the Lotus Pose, or stand on your head or perform some other asana, you will achieve nothing. The body has its own preferences, rigidities, suppleness. Listen to what your body is saying.

After every asana relax briefly and pay attention to what the body is telling you. Do you feel good? Was that stretch exhilerating? Are you in pain? Listen and act accordingly. A little pain (this might also be termed 'pleasurable pain') is inevitable in the beginning. Stop right there. If you pull a muscle too much, stop, and apply hot, wet compressess. Use a little soothing oil and massage the area. Be more cautious next time. Your muscles will inevitably get more elastic, the joints more supple, the bones stronger, if you practise steadily and regularly. The body that is stretched from top to toe, turned upside down in defiance of gravity, taught poise and balance and stability and calmness of mind will avoid physical and mental illness, the debilitating aspects of old age, and health and strength will be acquired. Biological age has nothing to do with linear age. Some young people have so degenerated, they have turned into walking cripples. Thwarted, frustrated and unhealthy, their imbalance and frustration is a danger to themselves and to the world.

With patience, steady, uninterrupted practice, and single-minded attention, the *sadhak* (the learner) changes himself, liberating his body and mind, restoring resonance and harmony to his life.

Three little stretching exercises
Do these before you begin a practice of asanas or any time during the day when you feel stiff and tired.

Standing stretch
Stand with the feet together and the arms at the sides. Inhale slowly and at the same time rise up on your toes and lift the arms above your head. Hold the breath in and stretch. Link your thumbs and stretch your arms as

though to touch the ceiling. Pull your body up and out from waist. Lift on to the very tips of your toes. Exhale and slowly lower the body and the arms to starting position. Repeat twice or more.

Lying stretch
Lie down on your back, with the feet together and the arms at the sides. Inhale and at the same time raise the arms slowly above your head to lie on mat. Retain breath and stretch. Link your thumbs and pull the arms up as far as possible, pulling up from the waist. Push the feet down as far as possible. Exhale and slowly lower the arms and bring the knees up to your chest. Hug the knees tightly to the chest with the arms and hold without breath for a few seconds. Inhale and slide the feet down to starting position. Bring the arms back to sides. Repeat twice or thrice.

Sitting stretch
Sit with the knees bent and the feet flat on floor. Clasp the hands *under* the thighs. Exhale and roll back, inhale and come up to a curled, sitting position, head on knees; exhale and roll back, inhale and come up. Rock back and forth, inhaling as you come up, exhaling as you go down, and keeping a tight hold of the under thighs. Do this several times, and massage kinks out of the back.

Benefits of all three simple stretching exercises are excellent. The stretch releases tension, the deep breathing brings in fresh supplies of oxygen to the blood, and the muscles and ligaments as well as the joints are subjected to a mild form of traction. Posture is improved and the body feels relaxed and relieved of stiffness and tension.

Another excellent exercise to fit into your day, whenever you have a little time, is to crawl around. Stand stiffly and put your hands on the floor. Walk on all fours but without bending your knees. Now bend your knees and crawl around on the carpet, making several rounds of the room till you feel tired. This tones up the abdominal organs and makes the legs very firm and shapely. It is excellent for slimming down bulges and protrusions all over the body.

Always finish with relaxation in the Corpse Posture or

Shavasana. Your body has been freshened, toned and stretched, and your mind too should now be in a reflective, relaxed state. Enjoy this wonderful feeling.

Yoga asanas for the over sixties
Figure 5:   Vajrasana (Diamond Posture)
Figure 8:   Baddhakonasana (Bound hands to feet posture)
Figure 9:   Dharmikasana (Devotional Pose)
Figure 11:   Sarvangasana (Shoulder Stand)
Figure 12 & 13:   Viparita Karani (Topsy–Turvy Pose)
Figure 14   (3) in Shirsh Asana (The Headstand)
Figure 18:   Bhujangasana (The Cobra)
Figure 20:   Matsyasana (The Fish)
Figure 21:   Vrikshasana (The Tree)
Figure 23:   Natrajasana (The Pose of the Dancing Shiva)
Figure 26:   Gomukhasana (The Cow-Face Posture)
Figures 27, 28 & 29:   Marichyasana (Spinal Twist)
Figure 31:   Halasana (The Plough)
Figure 32:   Salbhasana (The Locust)
Figure 33:   Dhanurasana (The Bow)
Figure 34:   Paripurna Shashasana (The Completed Hare)
Figure 35:   Ushtrasana (The Camel)
Figure 36:   Santulanasana (The Stretching Posture)
Figure 38:   Ananatasana (Vishnu's Couch Posture)
Not illustrated: Shavasana (The Corpse Posture)
Uddiyana, Nauli, Mula-Bandha and Ashwini Mudra should also be practised according to the instructions given. These are very important for maintaining the health of the sex glands and the urogenital area. Growing old is a process that occurs to every person. Doctors tell us that a linear decline begins after twenty to twenty-five years. With yoga you can stay youthful for ever with healthy muscles, strong bones, a good digestion and every gland working properly.

5.

RELAX THE YOGA WAY

Although the classic Yoga relaxation pose, Shavasana, was given at the end of the last chapter, many people find it impossible to relax if told to lie down on the floor and let themselves go. Instead, the body seems to tighten up, muscles are tensed, instead of relaxed and lactic acid is held within the tense muscles, producing stress and even pain.

What does it mean to relax? Most people don't really know what relaxation means. They say they are relaxing when watching a film or television, or driving for long hours to some picnic spot or beach, or amusing themselves by dancing in a disco or at a crowded party. However, the signs of tension are very apparent. Stiffness in the way the body is held, fidgeting, blinking rapidly, or a rigidly held head. They get headaches, digestive disturbances, insomnia, and chronic anxiety. Physical and mental endurance deteriorate and the capacity for work diminishes. They are edgy and irritable, and actively involved in pressures and tensions, which seem to be a major part of existence. To tell them to lie down and relax is worse than useless. They don't know how to relax or even what real relaxation means. An added drawback is that they are probably used to swallowing tranquillizers, analgesics, soporifics and all kinds of drugs which they hope will make them feel better.

Yoga offers a real solution to these problems. There are many different relaxation techniques in which the person is forced to take part, by visualization, by different breathing techniques and by active involvement, instead of simply lying down and trying to force the body and mind to relax. It is well worth trying out quite a few of them to see which works best for you. Yoga relaxation is a mind control of the nerves and the glandular system which controls the human body. The relaxation kriyas help to dissolve and remove the causes of stress. The centre of negative feelings is the hypothalamus in the brain which secretes a fluid which forces the adrenal glands into activity. Adrenalin squirts into the blood stream in a tense situation producing the *flight or fight* syndrome. Yoga deals directly with the stress centres by certain techniques which release tension and produce total freedom from both conscious and sub-conscious tensions.

Physical stress can change the heart rate and blood pressure, uric acid appears in the blood and ulcers, migraine headaches and stomach or muscle cramps can occur.

Much physical tension and stress, held in tight muscles and stiff spine, can be released through a practice of yoga asanas and deep breathing. The blood flow increases, oxygen is pumped through the blood and tension is released through the alternate stretching and relaxing of various parts of the body. If the mind is also concentrated on the movement, mental tension also diminishes. Short rests between asanas are necessary. Simply roll over on to the back or collapse into any tensionless pose to get relief from physical stress and exhaustion.

For really deep, profound relaxation, one must turn to the ancient relaxation techniques of yoga, where conscious tension is withdrawn and the body and mind are healed and restored as though in deep mediation. Sleep becomes an extension of deep relaxation instead of a restless, tension-filled period. In deep, relaxed sleep, cells are renewed and rebuilt and body emotions and the mind are calmed and rejuvenated, leading to positive good health. In Yoga relaxation the body's energy resources are conserved and renewed. Shavasana, the Corpse Posture, produces a relaxation state of roughly fifty-two per cent body tonus. Real relaxation begins when the body tonus falls below sixty per cent. Normal waking tension is around seventy per cent but when we sleep it should go down to thirty-eight per cent. Transcendental Meditation takes the body tonus down to about fifty-two per cent but real, deep relaxation as in yogic relaxation only begins below thirty-eight per cent. Below twenty-six per cent body tonus no one can live, but if one can get down to a relaxation state which is somewhere between thirty-eight per cent and twenty- six per cent then one is in a state of relaxation so deep that the body and mind repair themselves. A healing takes place which is of inestimable value to all those seeking not only relief from tension, but also a state of calm and peacefulness in which the mind is free to operate at maximum efficiency and the body is free from tension disturbances.

Constant stress can lead to all kinds of problems such as heart damage, ulcer formation and a lowered resistance to infection. Yogic relaxation employs much visualization which is not easy for many people. The relaxation techniques given here begin with more simple techniques in which muscles are used to tense and release stress, and continue on to where the mind takes over in deep relaxation techniques combined with breathing patterns and the use of sound or Mantras. As with all yoga techniques, pick and choose which of these work for you. Some will come easily, some you will find totally impossible and even unpleasant. There is nothing that says what you must or must not do. You have a choice. Try them for at least one week consecutively to give it a chance. None of the techniques are likely to be instantly successful. You have to first learn them properly and then put them into practise. In a yoga class it is much easier, because the teacher or guru will give you instructions as you lie passive on the floor, and you simply follow on with eyes closed. During a Yoga Nidra instruction class, I have seen at least twenty per cent of the class fast asleep before the completion of the whole process. Although sleep is not the aim of Yoga Nidra, the deep relaxation process had put tired bodies and mind into a withdrawal from stress and the natural outcome, for untrained students, was sleep.

For all yogic relaxation, concentration is necessary. The Zen No-mind state is excellent for this purpose. If your mind is churning round and round thinking of what to cook for dinner, what programme to watch on TV, or what your neighbour is doing in her garden, you will not succeed — the mind and the body work together for Yogic harmony. Many of the exercises in relaxation will begin with physical relaxation, but even so the mind must watch the whole process attentively.

Imagine the immense advantage of being able to relax at will. Office workers usually have their shoulders tensed, and the spine in an awkward position because there is not enough support for the back. Reading and examining pages of reports or files forces the ciliary muscles to remain tense for long periods of time, bringing on headaches which seem to be concentrated around the eyes. If you could simply take a few minutes off to lie down and relax, think how marvellously refreshed you would feel, as though you had experienced a long, refreshing sleep.

It is necessary, when you are beginning to relax, to prepare the conditions which will be favourable. A Yogi may be able to withdraw into himself and detach his mind and body from its surroundings, enjoying perfect peace and quiet, mind stilled, muscles relaxed, while still in the midst of a crowd. For the normal person this is not possible. Prepare your relaxation area carefully. I always prefer to lock myself into a room for both relaxation and meditation, with instructions that I am not to be called except for the most dire emergency.

When you are really relaxed then the blood pressure and heart beat and other body functions are at a state so reduced as simply to keep you alive. This allows you to be in a tension-less state which is very soothing and healing for the body and the emotions.

Follow these rules when you are starting to practise relaxation.

1. Always lie on a hard surface such as the floor with a thick carpet on top. Before going to sleep you may practise any favourite relaxation technique in bed, but you should do the real practice session on a folded rug or carpet on the floor.
2. Have your head facing north and your feet to the south, to take advantage of the earth's magnetic currents.
3. There should be no radio or TV in the room. Any sort of noise produces stress and distraction, and the body reacts negatively to this form of disharmony. When you are able to relax instantly, then noise may not disturb you, but for now, select a quiet place.
4. Pull a sheet or light rug over you if it is cool, since body temperatures will be lowered temporarily, when in relaxed state.
5. Do not wear anything tight around waist or neck as

nothing should restrict circulation or make you feel uncomfortable.

6. If you are uncomfortable lying on the floor (many people are) then put a pillow under your knees which will help the small of the back to lie flat against the floor.

7. Do not lie in the blazing sun on a beach or terrace for relaxation. Similarly, do not lie with the moon's light full on your face.

8. The room should be clean, airy, but darkened if possible. Draw the curtains to shut out light. Burning incense in the room often acts as a signal to prepare yourself for the relaxation process. You can work out other conditions which are helpful to you, personally.

9. Never get up suddenly or in a hurry — this could be not only counter-productive but dangerous.

10. Finally, remember to select (after at least one week of trial) those relaxation techniques which appeal to you and with which you feel most comfortable. For instance when I first learnt 'the Tingle', I was so pleased with the way I went almost instantly into a beautifully relaxed state, that I taught it to my daughter. She found it impossible and insisted that instead of relaxing as she was suppose to do, she kept feeling strange itches and shivers on her limbs and face. There is nothing in Yoga that says you must do this or that. Select your own favourite techniques, but first try them all and give them a fair chance to work. Some are more deeply relaxing than others. We will begin first with the light, as opposed to deep, relaxation techniques.

1. Watching the breath

Lie down, feet to the south and head to the north. Wriggle, squirm and stretch till you have released some tension from the muscles. Put a cushion under your knees if necessary and close your eyes. Keep your mind attentively on the body. Relax any tensions which are apparent to you. Are your shoulders hunched? Pull them down from your ears and let them lie loosely on the carpet. Is your neck tense, your teeth clenched, your eyes rigidly shut? Relax all of these tensions. Now begin slow rhythmic breathing. Keep to any count which feels comfortable but dispense with the held-in and held-out breaths. Simply breathe in to the count of six and out to the count of six. Do this consciously for some time till the rhythm is established and comes smoothly, on its own. Now watch the breath. Watch how it goes in through the nose and feels cool as you inhale. Watch it as you exhale, warm against the nostrils. Think of the sound OM as you breathe in and again OM as you breathe out. The word need have no special significance for you — simply regard it as a beneficial Mantra which acts powerfully on the mind and body. The breath should flow evenly in and out, in and out, till you are not only watching the breath but you yourself are the breath and there are no emotions, no tensions left in the body, only the breath, moving rythmically in and out, in and out. Relax and enjoy a state of bliss.

2.   *Inner light concentration*

Sit on your heels and bend forward till your head is on the mat in front of your knees in the posture known as Dharmikasana — the Devotional Pose (Figure 8). As already explained, this is a very tension-reducing pose because of the intense spinal stretch, relieving pressure on the spinal cord and brain. Your breath will be very light and shallow. Take your concentration into the point at which the head touches the floor and withdraw inward at this point. Now imagine your favourite colour — let it spread so that you are totally engulfed in this colour, as though you are floating in liquid colour. If you are relaxed you will feel as though you are a part of this colour into which a point of light will appear in the Third Eye area between your brows, known as the *Ajna Chakra*. Hold this light with passive attention. It might fade and return. Do not try to grasp or force it. Let it be. A marvellous feeling of relaxation will come about with this inner light experience. Often no light will appear. Do not be anxious or tense. Leave it alone. Simply continue to relax in this pose. Then breathe in deeply and sit up. Remain sitting for some time before getting to your feet again. The sense of relaxation should remain with you for some time.

3.   *Tension-cum-relaxation kriya*

Yoga kriyas often relieve tension and stress in the body by

first creating tension in the muscles before relaxing them. This is to use tension constructively in order to produce even greater relaxation. Lie down on your mat, head to the north and feet to the south. The arms and legs are comfortably apart, head tilted neither back nor forward but well positioned, as though in a standing position. Now take your attention down to the right foot. Tense the toes, curling them up, tense the foot back at the ankle, tense the whole leg up the knee, tighten the knee and keep it very stiff; now take this tension up the thigh, up and up to the buttock. Now feel the whole leg from toes to buttocks tight and tense. Hold this position as long as is possible. Now exhale slowly and begin releasing the tension from the buttock, slowly down over the leg till you reach the foot and then the toes. Relax and feel the whole leg from top to bottom relaxed. Repeat the same procedure on the other foot, inhaling as you tense up and exhaling as you relax.

Now inhale and begin tensing up the torso, starting with both buttocks and going slowly up from lower back and abdominal area to mid-back and waist, to upper back and chest and finally tensing both shoulders. Hold as long as possible and then slowly exhale and relax the tension from the top down, shoulders, upper back, and so on until you reach the buttocks. Relax.

Now begin to inhale again and tense the arms, beginning with the fingers, palms, wrists, forearms, upper arms and back to the shoulders. The hands should be tightly clenched into fists. Now exhale and release the tension from the top down, till the hands and fingers lie curled and relaxed, without tension.

Now inhale and begin to tense up the neck muscles, then the chin and jaw, up the sides of the face, screw up the eyes, tense the forehead muscles and the muscles of the head at the back. Hold for a few moments and then exhale slowly, releasing tension from the head down to the neck, opening and blinking eyes, relaxing the jaw, opening the mouth and feeling the tension run out, as it were. Breathe slowly and calmly and feel your body, from top to bottom, wholly relaxed. Because this is an active form of relaxation your mind has not had time to start churning around and worrying uselessly. It has been entirely occupied in following the movements of the body.

This is one relaxation technique which you can try in bed when you can't sleep. It can be repeated again and finally you may tense the whole body in one inhaled breath, from toes to head and relax on one exhaled breath from head to toes. For people who don't know how to relax, or don't know the difference between relaxation and tension, this is a very useful technique, before going on to more advanced ones.

4.   The tingle or recharging your batteries
Have you ever tried lying quietly and listening to your heart or pulse beats? It is not as impossible as it sounds. At first you can put your fingers lightly on any pulse spot: wrist, temples or your heart. Listen to the smooth, steady beat. Now lie back and let your body feel loose. Close your eyes. Concentrate on the pulse beating in your elbow (or wrist, or whichever is easy for you). Feel the steady throb like a small, but powerful battery charger. Shift your attention to some other part of the body where a pulse is beating. Move to the temples, the heart, the back of the knees, the wrist. Feel the tingle, the throb pulsing through your entire body. Try to take this behind your eyes, and then finally into the 'Third Eye' between the brows. Allow your concentration to end here. Feel the whole body vibrating gently, pouring new energy or *Shakti* into your body, relaxing you in a way you never thought was possible before. Relax and enjoy the feeling. Total relaxation will ensue.

5.   The nerve cleansers
There are a number of alternate nostril techniques in Pranayama which are used to balance the positive and negative forces in the body, thus bringing about a state of total release from mental tension. Because the technique is active and one is engaged in doing something, the mind is easily concentrated and the special breath pattern acts as a tranquillizer, first speeding up the breathing and then slowing it down to the point where only one breath is taken every minute. This in itself is extremely calming. When we are angry or upset, we breathe quickly, panting almost, in our distress. When we are calm the breath slows down to a steady rhythm. This form of breathing deliberately slows down the breath after speeding it up.

Sit in any straight-backed position and take in the first breath through the right nostril. Close off the right nostril with the thumb of the right hand and hold the breath briefly before exhaling through the left nostril. Shut off the left nostril with the little finger of the right hand and inhale through the right nostril. The breath comes in through the right nostril and is exhaled through the left nostril. First it may be done to a 6x3x6x3 rhythm and then faster to a 4x2x4x2 rhythm and then simply in from the right and out from the left with no pause at all till the breath is moving very rapidly in and out for about thirty rounds or more. Now reverse the rhythm. Begin to slow down the breath again, still taking it in from the right and out from the left, until the breath has been slowed down to 8x4x8x4, and then 10x5x10x5 and 12x6x12x6 and then even further if you are able to do it. Yogis can slow the breath down to a 64x32x64x32 count, taking in only one breath in three minutes. But this is for the adept practitioner and it is enough if you can slow the breath down to twice a minute. This breathing actually feeds the nerves, releasing tension and relaxing the entire nervous system as no tranquillizer can do.

6. Yoga Nidra — the psychic sleep of the Yogi
Many different versions of this relaxation technique are taught and I myself have learnt three different ones from three different teachers, but the best, and most effective, is undoubtedly the one taught by Dr Swami Gitananda of Ananda Ashram, Pondicherry. If we have some idea of what sleep means we can then understand the effectiveness of Yoga Nidra.

Most people pass through several stages of progressive sleep, alternating between states of dreaming and non-dreaming with four to seven periods of dreaming each night. Scientific experiments have shown that from the behavioural standpoint, the dream state appears to be a very deep level of sleep from which external stimuli are excluded. Slight noises, gentle touches, odours or any other stimuli, which would normally awaken a sleeper, pass unnoticed. If the depth of sleep is now measured by response to external stimuli then the dreaming state is a period of deep, deep, sleep.

From a physiological standpoint, however, the dreaming state is the lightest phase of sleep. Measured on the electroencephalograph it was shown that the activity of the brain was the same or even greater than when awake. The nerve-cells which provide a two-way communication between the brain and the body were discharging electrically at a rate that was a little faster than during wakefulness. The 'dreaming' brain was awake and so was the body, which showed a noticeable rise in heart rate, body temperature and respiration. The dream state is similar to a state of deep meditation or hypnosis where the individual, though awake, does not respond to external stimuli.

Yoga Nidra is a state in which slow-wave activity is present without the disturbances of Rapid Eye Movement sleep. It is a deeply relaxed state in which thoughts and dreams do not filter from the subconscious. 'In this state the individual is released back into the Universal or Cosmic State, but without memory consciousness.' Yoga Nidra provides the deepest state of relaxation of any of the Yoga relaxation techniques. It may be done either lying flat on the back or while sitting in a straight-backed yogic position. I prefer the lying down position since most people are conditioned to relax at least moderately, when they lie down.

It is necessary to make some preparation where Yoga Nidra is to be practised. In a Yoga class the doors will be closed and no one is allowed to enter or leave. The teacher gives his instructions in a soft, modulated voice. Except for his voice there is no sound, no disturbance of any sort. To be interrupted suddenly from the deep, deep Yogic sleep is dangerous. Jangled nerves, anxiety symptoms and increased tension will be the result.

Lie down on your back in as a relaxed position as possible. Your head should be to the north, your feet to the south. You may be uncomfortable on the floor, so put a small pillow under your knees to get the back flat. Start slow rhythmic breathing to a 8x4x8x4 count, which you should be very familiar with by now. Continue this form of breathing, allowing the body to become heavier and more relaxed. Now take the concentration into the solar plexus or what is known as the *Manipura Chakra* — the third of the psychic Chakras or centres in the body. (More will be said about this later.) From this area, imagine a point, small as a pin-head, from which you are about to direct an energy flow, first clock-wise and then anti-clockwise, breaking up the habit pattern of the nervous system by cutting across twelve nerve fields which emanate outwards from the solar plexus like numbers on a clock.

The circle is at first tight and small. Do not pay any attention to the breath, which will come and go rhythmically on its own. Concentrate on drawing, with your mind, slowly widening circles from this first small, tight one. Imagine, if you like, a pencil held in an imaginary hand. The first circle is drawn and then the pencil continues, spiralling outward, making progressively larger and larger circles, until finally the circle is large enough to enclose the entire body. First the spirals continue to go round and round in the solar plexus, gradually they spread to enclose the rib cage and the pelvis at top and bottom, then they continue until the top of the circle reaches the mid-chest and the bottom the upper thighs; then the top reaches the lower neck and middle thighs; then the circle reaches the chin and the shins, the eyebrows and the ankles, the tops of the head and the soles of the feet; finally take the spiral outside the head six inches (15 cms) above the top, and outside the feet, six inches (15 cms) below. Stop when the spiral reaches the outside of the top of the head. Relax with your consciousness settled at this point for half a minute or more. Now begin to spiral back into the body in a reversed anti-clockwise direction till you return to the point where you started in the solar plexus. Tighten the last circle down as though with a screwdriver into wood. The whole exercise should take about fifteen minutes.

Now relax into this deepest of all states of relaxation which has physical as well as psychic benefits. Continue to lie there, blissful and at peace, until the desire comes to move. Often there is the feeling that it is impossible to move — a catatonic-like state in which there is no desire to come out of this deeply restful state in which there is neither movement nor thought, and the mind and body are at peace as never before. There is no need to be afraid of not being able to move. The rested body will slowly shift and begin to come to life. Stretch, roll from side to side, and finally sit up very slowly. Never jump up and begin moving from this state of relaxation. Give the body a chance to benefit to the maximum from the state into which it has been. If this whole technique is done properly it is more relaxing than eight hours of sleep.

In addition to the deep relaxation this is a very rejuvenating process since the anabolic, regenerative process of cells is at the highest level and the nervous cell system is revived and strengthened. Insomnia will be a thing of the past and anxiety, fear, and depression cured. The whole body is repaired and given a real lift. Your body tonus will have fallen to the deepest relaxation level between thirty-eight per cent and twenty-six per cent.

It is wise to read the instructions carefully and visualize what you are going to do. First the relaxing, rhythmic breath, then the concentration into the solar plexus and then the tiny circle, widening and spiralling outward to enclose the entire body till it stops six inches (15 cms) above the head and six inches (15 cms) below the feet. Have a dry run, reading the instructions and following them bit by bit, without attempting the relaxation, until you are familiar with the whole process. Then lock yourself in your room, make sure you have at least half an hour to yourself, and go ahead and practise what might be the most important relaxation method you have ever tried.

Mini relaxation techniques to do throughout the day
1.   Lie down on a carpet or lie back in a comfortable chair. Close your eyes and let the body go limp. Consciously run the mind over from head to foot to locate any tense spots. Now imagine a scene which struck you at that time for its quiet beauty. A forest lane, a lonely seashore with the waves breaking gently against the beach, a mountain vista or a park filled with flowers. Choose your own scene and with your mind return there. Feel the wind, smell the flowers, the salt lick of the sea, the deep green of the forest. There is no one else there — only you. Enjoy the quiet sense of relaxation before breathing deeply and slowly sitting up.

2.   Sit back on your heels, with a straight spine and do ten rounds of the rhythmic breath. Perhaps you are now able to do the 10x5x10x5 rhythm or even

12x6x12x6. After ten rounds lie down on your back and close your eyes. Imagine that your mind is detached from your body and is floating above you in the air. Let it sail out through the window and high up over cities, mountains, seas, forest (this is an individual matter and must be centred around your own area). Now return, still winging through the air, till you are once again inside the body, which is lying on the floor as you left it. Sit up again on your heels and bend forward till your head touches the mat in front of your knees (Dharmikasana). Relax and feel a warmth start at the base of the spine and creep upwards into your head and your face. Behind the forehead, where the Third Eye is situated, feel the warmth. Sometimes at this stage colours like a rainbow flash before the eyes. Relax. Sit up slowly, breathe deeply and get up.

3. Lie down on the floor. Put a cushion under the knees. Relax the body as much as possible. Turn the head from side to side and wriggle and squirm till some tension is released from taut muscles. Now close your eyes. Start slow rhythmic breathing. With each breath feel warmth creeping up from the toes, up the ankles, knees, thighs, torso, neck and head. Feel it coming up through the fingers, hands, arms, shoulders and neck. The warmth is pleasing, like lying in a warm bath. The inner organs sink back and lose tension. Imagine darkness around the eyes. The eyeballs seem to drop back into the head. The earth seems to be pulling the body down, down till it is fused into the floor. The mind begins to move toward unconsciousness — it is still, free from past or present memories, and both body and mind are subject to healing, rejuvenating processes. Breathe deeply, stretch and sit up.

4. This is the No-Mind relaxation. Lie down on the floor and relax with rhythmic breathing. Now imagine a blank television screen in front of you. Your thoughts pass over this screen, which does not hold them but allows them to flow past. Soon the thoughts will cease and there will be only the empty screen. The mind has become empty like a canyon or a valley; the mind

becomes totally still. There is no separate identity now between you and the floor on which you are lying or the world around you. You are one with everything in a silence which knows no periphery nor centre, no movement, no depth nor height. It is just stillness of which you are a part. Breathe deeply, stretch and sit up very slowly. Feel refreshed and invigorated, calm and ready to face anything.

5. Let's go back to Exercise 1 in which you have imagined yourself in a park filled with flowers, or on a wind-swept beach or in a green, green, forest lane. Imagine you are there once again but this time think of all the details. What did you see, how did you feel? What were the colours like of the sky, the trees, the sand? Picture all this vividly, feel yourself there, in that space and when this is accomplished bring that area with you into any stressful situation. When you feel tense, nervous, worried, upset, take yourself into your forest, beach or park. Project it around you as a shield. This is not a yogic technique but one which was thought up by a psychologist who taught it to prison inmates and found they were more calm, less inclined to go into rages or into fits of depression. It is called 'Create A Space'.

Most relaxation exercises are aimed at producing physical tension-free states and internal quiet and balance. Think of the enormous benefits of moving the attention from work (and worry!) to something which relaxes the body and quietens the mind — a prelude, as it were, to deeper states of meditation.

Meditation is also a form of relaxation and in fact Transcendental Meditation aims at just that — to create a sense of total relaxation in which the mind is emptied and the ego displaced. Masks, defences, preconceptions and opinions fall away and dissolve and there is nothing left but 'a pearly radiance'. In this void, one's true nature is reborn. In meditation, as in deep relaxation, the heart slows down and anxiety and external pressures of the world are reduced. Body and mind, in these states, are subjected to strong healing influences. The right hemisphere of the brain is activated, increasing latent powers and subconscious knowledge. Creative talent is enhanced.

When you have practised relaxation of various kinds for some time, then try a little meditation. There is nothing very esoteric about meditation, although there are hundreds of different kinds — the paths are different but the final goal is the same. Here are two simple but extremely effective techniques which anyone can try.

Meditation in god's hour

This is a very simple but very effective technique which is carried out only in the early hours of the morning, roughly one hour before dawn, when the world still sleeps and destructive thoughts and noises have not begun to pollute the atmosphere.

Sit quietly, back straight, hands folded in lap, facing north or east. Allow the mind to become quite still. Breathe quietly and be aware of the breath moving in and out of the lungs. The mind should be quiet but aware, waiting. In Zen there is a saying about meditation: 'Sitting quietly, doing nothing; spring comes and the grass grows again.' Sit quietly, doing nothing. Let your thoughts come and go. Don't hold on to them. Feel the quietness of the morning seeping into your mind, your nerves, your bones and your very skin. Soon you will find yourself in a state where you can see there is no real edge to anything, only an endless inter-penetration of the universe of which you are a part. You and the rest of mankind are seen as an integral part of the environment, one aspect of the whole intricately balanced organism of the natural world. Positive and negative principles are in dynamic balance. You feel a state of serene detached awareness of eternal things, an aloofness, impersonal yet benign. When it is time to give up, you will come out of this state on you own. Don't move for some time. Keep the serene feeling with you as long as possible. Stretch and come back to the everyday world.

Approach to the cave

For those who find passive meditation difficult here is an active form which can be very effective. In this you use intuitive and subsurface powers which are normally submerged by the noise of the mind or by the automatic reactions of the mind. Sit quietly in any of the straight-backed sitting positions of Yoga. Imagine that you are walking and approaching a long tunnel-like cave. Imagine the walk, meandering through woods, fields and meadows. There are flowers and green grass and rippling streams. Enjoy all of this in detail since it is you who are creating the scene. Nothing in it will be objectionable to you. Everything is pleasant and enjoyable. You approach the mouth of the cave which is dark. You know that inside, at the very end of the cave, is something or someone who is waiting to see you. You approach slowly and ask one question. The thing or person in the Cave will answer you, if not after the first time then on succeeding attempts.

In this meditation, the mind, concentrating on something specific, cannot involve itself in worries and anxieties. The answer you are waiting for will be your own answer from your subconscious Self which is waiting to communicate with you when the 'mind screens' are knocked off. Since every human being has access to all kinds of material within, when the conscious filters or barriers are removed you are in touch with your subconscious or what Brunton terms the *Overself*.

Learning how to relax could be the most important thing you could teach yourself. Real relaxation releases tension from body, emotions and mind, as well as tensions which have accumulated in the subconscious mind. These techniques can help you to lead a healthier, less stressful and more serene life as well as a more creative one. Relaxation, like breathing and Yogic asanas, has a rejuvenating effect on body and mind as well as on the glands, organs and nerves. Half an hour or more each day should be devoted to one or more of these practices. The effects are nothing short of miraculous.

And now, finally, let us learn how to polarize the body with polarity kriyas — a process which combines breathing techniques, visualization and deep relaxation. Yogic union cannot exist without polarity of the negative and positive forces in the body, an energy flow that stabilizes body and mind, regulating the 'electric flow in the nervous system and the ionization of cellular energy'. Yoga believes that man possesses five bodies: the Physical Body (Annamaya Kosha), the Vital Body (Pranayaya Kosha), the Memory and Conscious Body (Manomaya Kosha), the Super Conscious Mind Body (Vijnanamaya

Kosha), and the Cosmic Body (Anandamaya Kosha). If these five bodies of man are not properly aligned with each other from lack of real polarity, then depression, disease and accidents occur. If we breathe correctly, that is if we practise slow, deep breathing, then electrolytic balance in the body is maintained. With shallow breathers the polarity begins to degenerate and negative emotions and destructive tendencies occur. This simple technique will restore polarity to the body, make the emotions healthy and stable and the mind and body in perfect harmony. Accident-prone people should do this polarity Kriya regularly since accidents that constantly happen — cutting yourself with a knife, banging your head on the door jamb as you walk through, slipping and falling when there is seemingly nothing to slip on — all these could be due to a malalignment of the Panch Koshas or Five Bodies of Man.

Anu-loma-viloma Kriya (Polarity Kriya)
Lie down on your back in Shavasana, with your head to the north and feet to the south. In this kriya this position is very important in order to take advantage of the magnetic current which flows from north to south. Your room should be well ventilated and there should be quiet and peace with no disturbances to jangle the nerves. Begin deep rhythmic breathing to the 8x4x8x4 count. Take in the breath for a count of 8, hold the breath in for a count of 4, exhale for a count of 8 and hold the breath out for a count of 4. When your breathing has settled smoothly into this rhythm then imagine or visualize the breath as coming from the top of the head and flowing out of the feet as you inhale. Most students have problems with this since one is accustomed to breathe first in the abdominal area and then mid-chest and then the high clavicular area. This breath however, in a calm relaxed state can be visualized. Inhale and imagine the breath pouring down slowly over the body and out at the feet. Exhale and feel the breath moving up over the body and out over the top of the head. You should breathe in to a count of 8 as the breath sweeps down from the head to outside the feet. Suspend the breath for a count of 4, exhale as the breath sweeps up from the feet and suspend the breath for a count of 4. Now picture the inhaled breath to have a warm golden colour

and the exhaled breath to have a cool, silvery-blue colour. Sweep these two breaths back and forth over the body, until the body settles into a deeply relaxed state. You may imagine that the sound of sounds, OM, is wafted back and forth through the body with the breath for powerful, healing and restoring effects. The relaxation that comes with this kriya is deep and conscious relaxation. The polarity of the body is restored and energy conserved and built up into a powerful storehouse for later use.

Do not jump up from this polarity kriya or be in a hurry to take up your normal activities again. Lie quietly, enjoying the blissful sense of relaxation. Do not allow your thoughts to wander off into normal activity. Keep the mind blank — enjoy a deep sense of total mind/body relaxation. Stretch, breathe and stretch again and slowly sit up.

This relaxation technique may be done at the end of the yoga asanas or by itself. Do it consciously and with the mind attentively following every part of the technique. If your mind wanders off on its own, the effects of this polarity kriya will be lost. If it is properly done then physically, mentally, emotionally and spiritually, you will have enormous benefits. Very often, the first time is not successful. Be patient. Next time you will have more success. Yoga is not for those who are impatient or want quick results. Results will surely come with the right practice.

6.

HOW TO LIVE A YOGA LIFE

Having read so far you are probably wondering how to incorporate a full yoga programme into your daily life. You are a busy person and simply haven't the time to do everything that is recommended in this book. If this is your reaction then your priorities are wrong and your life style needs changing. If you want to reap the benefits of yoga you need to devote some time every day to it. One hour in the morning and another hour, or half-hour, in the evening is the minimum. Most people practising yoga make it a point to get up early at the hour before dawn, which is 'Brahma Murtha' or 'God's hour', for meditation. If you don't get up before dawn you can at least wake one hour earlier than you usually do and utilize this best of all times for yoga. There are however, some people whose metabolism is such that they stay awake late at night and wake late each morning. Adjust your schedule to your own convenience, although if you were to come for instruction to an ashram, you would be forced to get up in the very early hours of the morning to fit in the entire yoga programme.

The new interest in yoga, which started about twenty years ago, seems to have spread to even the most remote parts of the world and especially throughout Europe and America. This has forced a certain change in traditional yoga and new dimensions have been added to the original teachings. The interaction between western students and the ancient system of yoga has resulted in more down-to-earth goals for the aspirant. Instead of Moksha — liberation from the cycle of rebirths — the western student of yoga is interested in the more specific and tangible goals of a healthy body, supple and flexible joints, a smooth-working glandular system, and a mind and emotions that are controlled, and not subject to stresses and strains. In fact what is being sought after is a way to live happier, healthier lives without recourse to drugs and dangerous medicines. The developing interaction between the thoughts and philosophies of the East and the more pragmatic approach of the West, has interesting repercussions in the teaching of Yoga. Easterners tend to accept more easily, Westerners question everything, although there are today thousands and thousands of young people from the West who have handed over their minds to one of the Gurus with unquestioning, zombie-like faith. But these are a different crowd: disillusioned young people from affluent countries who are not prepared to go through the strenuous disciplines of yoga, but who seek an easy escape from their own frustrations.

Those who come to learn yoga are the more intelligent, higher beings, seeking a philosophy and a process which will evolve human beings into more integrated personalities so that real harmony of body and mind can prevail.

If we return to Chapter II which deals with diet, you will have realized that you cannot continue to eat as you have been doing and expect good results. The body and mind are very dependent on the food which supples nutrients, vitamins and all the other necessary factors which make the difference between good and bad health. Over-eating is one of the most common evils in today's world, leading to the diseases connected with ageing: cancer, late onset diabetes, arthritis, heart and vascular disease and senility.

The fallacy that the body needs three or four good meals a day in order to keep it going is just that: a fallacy. Up to the age of twenty, the body needs plenty of health-giving foods to build it up and provide a solid base for health. After that, *the less you eat the better*. Does this sound surprising? There are hundreds and thousands of yogis, fit and looking half their age, who eat very sparingly and only once or twice a day. Dr Roy Walford of the UCLA School of Medicine has presented his discoveries about ageing in his book *Immunological Theory of Ageing* , which is recognized as a significant contribution to the theory of the ageing process. Dr Walford discovered that immune dysfunction causes ageing and that the weakening of the immune system (the body's primary stress filter) leads to 'disease susceptibility and acceleration of the ageing processes leading to death'. If the immune system was strengthened and prevented from deteriorating, then the natural decay process was slowed, and it could be accomplished by *dietary restriction*. Dr Walford discovered in his experiments that the immune system deteriorated when the thymus gland (which produced a hormone called Thymosin) started to cease proper functioning. The ageing process was slowed down by treating the patient with artifically extracted thymosin but it also slowed down when *caloric intake was restricted*. When less food was eaten the thymus seemed to function better and longer. The thymus begins to decay just after puberty, increasing stress and decreasing the body's ability to deal with this stress, with resulting ageing of the body and mind. According to Walford the chief means of preventing immune failure and preserving youth is 'a habitual, lifelong adherence to a low calorie diet which offers adequate minerals and vitamins'. The statement 'lifelong adherence to a low calorie diet' should make everyone consider his own eating habits. Instead of a tall glass of milk, two eggs and bacon, toast with butter, coffee, juice and perhaps cereal for breakfast, an healthy alternative would be a small glass of fruit juice, a slice of brown bread with perhaps a poached egg, and one piece of fruit. A restricted low calorie diet is one in which a person eats no more than fifteen times his normal, lean body weight. This diet should consist of the 'broadest range of foods possible as well as a multi-vitamin tablet'. A person should eat well but never in excess. If the yoga diet of fifty per cent raw fresh foods, twenty-five per cent yogurt, cottage cheese, buttermilk and milk, and twenty-five per cent cooked foods such as cereals, vegetables, legumes and beans, is followed then the person is eating wisely and well. Many people are under the impression that if their diet is vegetarian then they are eating in a healthy and nutritious way. They couldn't be more wrong: many 'junk foods' are vegetarian. Refined carbohydrates, butter and cream, fried foods, ice-cream and pastries are all vegetarian and every one is harmful. Cokes, tea and coffee are also extremely harmful to the system. A diet which is light, nutritious and wholesome, with plenty of fresh fruit and vegetable juices, whole fruits and raw vegetables, should be followed. In most Indian ashrams only two meals are served: one in the morning and the next in the early evening, before sunset. If, however, you plan to eat three or four meals a day, see that your lightest meal is at night.

Pranayama or deep breathing should also be a part of your daily routine. Combined with the asanas it keeps muscles stretched and limber. Tight muscles limit the flexibility of the skeleton and put extra strain on the cartilage and ligament structures. Asanas will soon teach you to move rhythmically and smoothly like a cat.

Relaxation follows on and combines with diet, breathing to slow down the ageing process which is so dependent on the healthy functioning of the glands, and the digestive system.

But how can you work all this in to a daily routine? At the end of this book you will find a twelve-week programme for asanas, pranayama and relaxation. It is not necessary to follow it rigidly since yoga is the antithesis of rigidness. Use it as a guide to help you incorporate yoga into your life, to make it an integral part of your whole existence. When you get up in the morning, stretch while you are still in bed. Raise your arms high above your head and stretch. Breathe and stretch, first on your back and then on either side. Don't allow your mind to begin worrying about what is going to happen during the day. Sit up slowly and then get up. Do the stretching exercise standing, three times.

Now drink a small glass of fresh fruit juice, or a cup of herbal tea, or a glass of warm water with lemon juice and honey. All these are an excellent start to the day and will encourage peristaltic activity so that you do not suffer from constipation.

Before starting a practice of asanas you should empty your bowels and bladder, clean your teeth, and wash or have a bath. A warm shower is fine but don't soak in a hot bath before a practice of yoga. Wear clean, loose clothes, the absolute minimum in the summer, but you may need something warm in the winter. Now follow the chart and begin your practice. Keep your mind attentively on what you are doing. You will discover an extended awareness, a more perceptive appreciation of yourself and others as you proceed with your regular practice.

If you are trying to lose weight, do not eat for thirty minutes to one hour after your yoga practice so that your metabolism which was speeded up, remains high. In that half hour, move around, do a bit of gardening or dusting or something which needs a little movement.

Eat a healthful breakfast. Do not stuff yourself with fried foods and white bread. See how much better you feel when you eat well. Your eating habits will change as you grow more conscious and aware of the beauty and intricacy of your own body.

During the day, try to practise one or two mini-relaxation techniques. Breathe the rhythmic way when you have five minutes to spare. Practise the tightening and relaxation of the anal muscles (Mula–Bandha and Ashwini Mudra) as often as possible during the day. Since these can be done while standing, sitting or lying down with no-one any the wiser, it is a good idea to do them several times a day.

Lunch should be light and refreshing and try to follow it with a brief relaxation period. Perhaps you have by now perfected some technique which puts you into a relaxed state very quickly. If not, simply lie flat and let your muscles grow heavy. At the end of a long day, do not relax with a cup of coffee and a cigarette or with a scotch and soda. That is not true relaxation. Do a few stretching and limbering asanas. Try the inverted, upside-down asanas to relax tired and stiff muscles. Have a bowl of yogurt and some fresh fruit or a blender shake made from fruit juices, brewer's yeast and honey.

Before your light supper, do ten minutes' meditation. Then try a more lengthy relaxation kriya such as Yoga Nidra or the Polarity Kriya. Go to bed by ten o'clock if possible. Yogis believe that the earth's radiation is best at this time for sound sleep. Soon, after a modified regime such as this you will find your weight has adjusted itself, your digestive system will be working smoothly and your taste, vision, touch, sense of smell and calmness will have been heightened. You will enjoy life more, be able to do more, and accomplish more. It is a good idea to get out for a walk or swim in the evenings or on weekends. Use the rhythmic breath when you walk, counting an even 6x6x6x6 — breathe in for six steps, out for six, in for six, out for six, or add a held-in and held-out breath again for a count of six. This way you will double the benefits of a walk in the open, as well as filling your body with prana and energy.

There is, of course, much, much more to yoga than what we have touched on in this book but for that you will need a guru. Until then you can revolutionize your whole life, stop the ageing process or at least slow it down, while retaining all your faculties till the day you die. This alone should make it worthwhile to learn Yoga.

How many of us have known friends, relatives, or acquaintances who have grown old and senile, lying in bed unable to control their natural functions, with broken or stiff bones that do not allow any movement — a burden and sorrow to those who look after them, and a terrible tragedy for themselves. Is this the necessary corollary to growing old?

No, says yoga: stay fit and healthy until the day you die. A yoga teacher under whom I once studied, always told us at some point during the class that breath was life and when a yogi died, he allowed himself to stop breathing. When the breath was stopped long enough, death came. It always struck me as a very beautiful notion and a very beautiful way to die.

When you have practised the asanas, learnt the special breathing techniques and taught yourself how to relax, you will have made a distinct change in your body, mind and emotions. The correct diet too is of the utmost importance. There will be many beneficial changes in your health and your general outlook on life. You will be slimmer, more supple, flexible and without stiffness. You will have learnt how to relax and deal with strains and tensions with a calm, detached mind. Choose the asanas, kriyas and mudras which are suitable to your body needs. The same asanas are not always the right ones. You will have learnt to listen to what your body is saying and follow its instructions. You will *feel* the difference between a practice which is yogic, bringing harmony, and one which is destructive and wasteful of energy.

After a certain age the body has areas of stiffness, muscle cramps, inflexibilities of joints, and even aches and pains in certain areas. On those days, take it easy. Do some extra pranayama, balance and stretching asanas, and lots of relaxation. Perhaps the body has stored up lactic acid in the muscles, causing stiffness. Breathing will help as fresh, oxygenated blood circulates through the body. The charts and programme for ten weeks given in the next chapter are meant only as a guide, there is nothing inflexible about them. You are free to make up your own programme. Try always to combine forward bends, with backward bends. If the posture forces the body in one way then immediately afterwards a posture to balance the first one should be done. For instance, the Plough is well followed by Paschimottanasana — the forward stretching pose. The Cobra which uses the body from the waist up, is usually followed by the Locust in which the lower half of the body below the waist is exercised.

As you become more and more supple and more and more expert, try out some of the more difficult asanas. They will add a new dimension to your practice. In six months' time you should be a changed person, both mentally and physically. Remember that Yoga means union, oneness, and all the aspects of diet, breathing, asanas and relaxation go together, for maximum benefit. One hour of practice each day is ideal. Breathing techniques and relaxation can be done in addition, perhaps during the quiet evening hours. For those who are retired and senior citizens, even more time may be devoted to learning and reading and practising this wonderful discipline. No one is ever too old for Yoga.

7.

TEN-WEEK PROGRAMME FOR BEGINNERS

First week

1. Begin with the Standing stretch and do it three times. Now sit in Vajrasana (Figure 4) and do the sectional breathing — first abdominal, then mid-chest and then clavicular; do each one separately, three times each. Now combine all three into one complete yoga breath. Pay conscious attention to the breath and breathe in and out rhythmically six times.

2. Bend forward into Dharmikasana (Figure 8) and relax into this tension-relieving posture. Now roll forward and do the Paripurna Shashasana (Figure 34) three times.

3. Do the two parts of the Vyagrahasana (Figures 2 and 3) at least six times or more to help you build strong abdominal muscles and teach correct abdominal breathing.

4. Do Matsyasana (Figure 20) with legs crossed easily, if the Lotus Pose is too difficult. Breathe deeply in the mid-chest area.

5. Stand up and do the balance poses of Vrikshasana (Figure 21) and Natrajasana (Figure 23).

6. Lie down on your back and do Shavasana, the Corpse posture with some deep rhythmic breathing. Release tension consciously from muscles that have been pulled and flexed beneficially. Close your eyes and watch the breath. Take at least five minutes for this deep relaxation before sitting up and beginning the day's work. In the evening you may do some more stretching postures and one or two of the breathing techniques followed by a favourite relaxation technique.

Second week

1. Do the standing stretch three times. Sit in Vajrasana (Figure 4) and do some Bellows breathing, bending forward as the breath is expelled in short 'whooshes'. This is a cleansing breath which lowers the carbon dioxide level in the blood. It is a good way to start a yoga practice.

2. Still sitting in Vajrasna, practise abdominal, mid-chest and clavicular breathing, each one separately, three times. Now practice the Complete Yoga breath, putting the three sections together and using Aaaah, Ooooo, and Mmmmm as vibratory adjuncts to the exhaled breath.

3. Lie down on your back and do the Uttanapadasana (Figure 37), first one leg at a time and then both together. Do each a minimum of three times.

4. From Uttanapadasana (Figure 37) carry on into Halasana (Figure 31) trying for a greater stretch each time. Repeat three times.

5. Turn over on your face and try Bhujangasana (Figure 18) three times followed by Bhujangi Kriya three times.

6. Still lying on your face, do Salbhasana (Figure 32), the Locust posture, which should follow the Cobra. Do each leg three times separately and then both legs together.

7. Sit up and attempt two of the sitting postures: Siddhasana (Figure 5) and the difficult Baddhakonasana (Figure 7). Remember to 'butterfly' the knees to get them supple.

8. Do Matsyasana (Figure 20), trying to get a real arch into the spine and the head forced radically backward.

9. Do the Vyaghrahasana (Figures 2 and 3) and try to get a very high arch into the spine on the exhaled breath.

10. Relax in Shavasana and do some rhythmic breathing or any of the shorter relaxation techniques such as The Tingle. Between asanas take short rests on your back or in any relaxed posture.

Third week
1. Do the standing stretch three times and sit in Vajrasana (Figure 4) and do some deep breathing to the rhythm of 4x2x4x2 and then 6x3x6x3 and on to 8x4x8x4.

2. Lie down on your back and attempt the Shoulder Stand, Sarvangasana (Figure 11). Get someone to help you if it is difficult.

3. Try the Half-shoulder Stand, Viparita Karani (Figures 12 and 13), fanning the legs back and forth to activate the pancreas. Hold the pose with deep abdominal breathing for as long as possible.

4. Attempt the walk-up to the Headstand, Shirshasana (Figure 14). It is enough to get into the inverted posture with your feet still on the floor (Figure 3). Hold this pose with deep, slow breathing for as long as possible.

5. Try the inverted Japanese Bridge, Vilomasana (Figures 16 and 17), both with hands under shoulders and later with hands in the prayer position.

6. Do the Fish Pose, Matsyasana (Figure 20) and get a really high arch into the back. Hold it a few seconds longer every time.

7. Stand up and do the sideways stretching pose, Parsvakonasana (Figure 39) Repeat each side three times.

8. Complete your practice with a deep relaxation technique — pick one and keep to the same one for a whole week.

Fourth week
1. Do the standing stretch three times. Sit in Vajrasana (Figure 4) and do first the Bellows breath through the mouth and then complete yogic breathing with the OM sound of Aaaaa, Oooooo, Mmmmmmm.

2. Bend forward from Vajrasana into Dharmikasana (Figure 8) and relax with shallow breathing, visualizing your favourite colour. After two or three minutes roll over into Paripurna Shashasana (Figure 34). Then repeat the roll and sit up three times. Pay attention to the breath.

3. Do the Shoulder Stand (Figure 11) and retain the pose with abdominal breathing for as long as possible.

4. Do Matsyasana (Figure 20) and repeat three times or hold for one minute.

5. Do Halasana (Figure 31) and try to get a really good stretch. Follow with Paschimottanasana, the forward stretch (Figure 19). Don't worry if you can't touch your toes. Hold on to ankles or even shins.

6. Do Gomukhasana (Figure 26) once on either side, holding for at least thirty seconds. Do the lateral spinal twists of Marichyasana (Figures 27, 28, 29) repeating each posture twice on either side. Keep your breathing slow and deep.

7. Relax after this strenuous workout. Lie in Shavasana (Figure 40) and do any of the visualization techniques which induce a feeling of calmness and peace.

Fifth week
1. Do the standing and lying stretches. Follow with any breathing technique while sitting in Vajrasana (Figure 4). Attempt the alternate nostril breathing today. Watch the movements of the fingers and the breath closely.

2. Today try the complete Headstand (Figure 14) Be very careful and have someone stand near you to see you

don't fall. Hold for only ten seconds and roll down. Lie down and relax.

3. Do the Shoulder Stand (Figure 11). Hold for at least thirty seconds. Go into Viparita Karani (Figures 12 and 13) and fan legs back and forth before holding position for thirty seconds.

4. Do the Fish posture (Figure 20) and hold for at least thirty seconds, with deep mid-chest breathing.

5. Sit up and then kneel and backbend into Ushthrasana (Figure 35), repeating it only once. If you can't hold your heels, simply backbend and let the arms dangle.

6. Lie down and do leg lifts — front, side and back. First do Uttanapadasana (Figure 37) with one leg at a time and then both legs. Turn over on to the left side and do Anantasana (Figure 38), holding the position for as long as possible. Roll over on your face and do Salbhasana (Figure 32) with one leg and then with both legs. Roll over on your right side and repeat Anantasana (Figure 38). Relax with some deep rhythmic breathing on your back.

7. Stand up and attempt the Hand to foot Posture (Figure 24), three times on either side. Hold on to something if you overbalance.

8. Try any of the sitting postures including Padmasana (Figure 6), the famous Lotus posture. Try it with one leg at a time and attempt to get the knee right down.

9. Relax in Shavasana (Figure 40) and do some rhythmic breathing to slow down the body.

Sixth week
1. Do the standing and lying stretches three times each. Sit in Vajrasana (Figure 4) and do the Aaaa, Oooo, Mmmm breathing for six to ten times.

2. Stand up and do the balance posture Vrikshasana (Figure 21) and repeat with both sides, holding,

without teetering for as long as possible.

3. From Vrikshasana, bend your knee and do the Vatsyayuasana (Figure 22). This needs very flexible knees and leg joints. Do not force the posture. Support yourself with your hands in the beginning.

4. Try the beautiful Vamadevasana (Figure 25). In the beginning it is enough to simply get the legs in the right positions flat on the mat. This is a very intense stretch so take it easy.

5. Do Shirshasana (Figure 14) and hold the pose for up to twenty seconds. Roll down and relax on your back.

6. Do Salbhasana (Figure 32) followed by Bhujangasana (Figure 18) followed by Dhanurasana (Figure 33). These three poses exercise in turn first the area above the waist, then the area below the waist and finally both parts simultaneously. Flexibility and suppleness are increased tremendously.

7. If you feel brave enough try Rajkapotasana (Figure 30). Don't hurry: you have all the time in the world to do these asanas. There is never any hurry in yoga. If not today, then do them tomorrow or some other time.

8. Practise some of the sitting postures again, aiming for a good firm, straight-backed posture. Try Virasana (Figure 10) which exercises the knees and toes.

9. Lie down and do the Polarity Relaxation technique, if you have enough time. Relax, unwind.

Seventh week
1. Do both sitting and lying stretches. Sit in Vajrasana (Figure 4) and do the Bellows Breath first through the mouth and then through the nose. Do the complete yogic breathing ten times.

2. Stand up and practise Uddiyana Bandha and Nauli if you can. These two should be done *every day* from

now on. Practice Mula–Bandha and Ashwini Mudra three times a day. Just because these contractions are so simple to do, don't minimize their effects: they are powerful.

3. Do the Headstand (Figure 14). Hold for at least one minute or longer.

4. Do the Shoulder Stand (Figure 11) and hold for up to three minutes. Concentrate on keeping the breath in the abdominal area and the chin pressed tightly into the sternum to activate the thyroid.

5. Do the Fish (Figure 20) to release tension on the neck area after the Shoulder Stand.

6. Do Halasana (Figure 31) and follow up with an opposite stretch, Paschimottanasana (Figure 19).

7. Do Salbhasana (Figure 32) and follow with the Cobra (Figure 18) and Dhanurasana (Figure 33).

8. Practise the important Baddhakonasana (Figure 7) which prevents urinary troubles and has a rejuvenating effect on the sexual organs. It also acts as a mood elevator. Try and sit in this posture for one minute Roll over and relax.

9. Practise all three of the spinal twists one after the other (Figures 27,28,29). Make sure you are following instructions carefully and your mind is attentively following every move and every breath that you take.

10. Relax in Shavasana and do some deep rhythmic breathing for at least ten minutes.

Eighth week
1. Start with the standing and lying stretches and massage the spine and warm it up with the sitting (rocking) stretch.

2. Sit in Vajrasana (Figure 4) and bend over into Dharmikasana (Figure 8). Roll over into Paripurna

Shashasana (Figure 34) and repeat three times.

3. Do Vilomasana (Figures 16 and 17) and then the higher arched Chakrasana (Figure 15).

4. Do Sarvangasana (Figure 11) and Halasana (Figure 31), followed by Paschimottanasana (Figure 19). These are all excellent spinal stretches to give you a strong and supple spine. A healthy spine is a healthy body is the yogic saying.

5. Do the Headstand (Figure 14) and hold it for one minute while you practise Mula–Bandha and Ashwini Mudra in this inverted posture. If you cannot do the Headstand because of any limitation, substitute the Shoulder Stand (Figure 11) and the walk-up to the Headstand.

6. Do some of the more difficult postures such as Vamadevasana (Figure 25) and Rajkapotasana (Figure 30).

7. Sit in any of the classical sitting postures and do some deep, slow rhythmic breathing. Try the 10x5x10x5 count and the even slower 12x6x12x6 count.

8. Relax into Shavasana (Figure 40) and do any of the deep relaxation techniques which you have learnt. Stay relaxed for a minimum of ten minutes before you sit up and resume your everyday life. Make sure when you are relaxing that no interruptions or noise jangles your nerves. It could be dangerous.

Ninth week
1. You should now be reasonably familiar with all the asanas and the breathing techniques.
   Begin your ninth week with the usual stretches and then do extra pranayama for the first, third and fifth days of the week. Start with the Bellows breath and do this from Vajrasana (Figure 1) at least three times to rid the blood of carbon dioxide.

2. Now do the three-part complete yoga breath, trying to

get the breathing very smooth like a wave. After five deep, complete breaths, begin the vibratory breathing with Aaaa for abdominal area, Ooooo for the mid-chest area and Mmmmmm for the clavicular area. As you breath in, think the sounds; as you breathe out, sound them loudly. Do this for at least another five rounds.

3. Practise the Ujjayi breath. This is energy-renewing and also excellent for tonsils or throat complaints. Do it at least five times.

4. Finish with ten rounds of rhythmic breathing trying to slow down the breathing gradually until you can do a 12x6x12x6 count easily.

5. Now do some of the inverted postures: The Head-stand (Figure 14), Viparita Karani (Figures 12 and 13), Sarvangasana (Figure 11), and Chakrasana (Figure 15).

6. Do Matysyasana (Figure 4) Paschimottanasana (Figure 19), Baddhakonasana (Figure 7) and Vilomasana (Figures 16 and 17). All these exercises, as well as the inverted postures, are gland stimulators. The quality of your hair, skin, teeth, internal muscles, as well as the health of your ovaries, prostate gland, vas deferens and urinary system are largely dependent on the good healthy working of the endocrine gland system, the adrenal glands and the thyroid and parathyroid. Gonadal stimulation leads to strong and healthy sex organs. Above all, when the glands are working properly there is vitality, youthful good looks, and a supple, resilient body.

7. Relax into Shavasana (Figure 40) and do any of the visualization techniques to calm down the nervous system. Take at least ten minutes after the end of your practice, which was extensive. During the week, it is not necessary to do every asana every day. Pick and choose, and if you have less time then do fewer asanas but do them slowly and thoroughly. Never rush through, thinking you will benefit. Yoga needs careful

attention, slow, smooth movements, rest between strenuous asanas. Take it easy. You will get much greater benefits by a slow and careful approach than by a hurried, frantic one.

Tenth week

1. Stretch. Always begin your practice with stretches combined with deep breathing. You may stretch and twist up, down and sideways.

2. Do some rhythmic breathing while sitting in Vajrasana (Figure 4) and then again lying down. Try the Ujjayi breathing for about five minutes. Do some alternate nostril breathing.

3. Do the Shoulder Stand (Figure 11) and follow it with the Plough (Figure 31). Do Matsyasana (Figure 20) and remember that the Fish should always follow the Shoulder Stand and the Plough.

4. Now do the forward stretch Paschimottanasana (Figure 19) and follow up with the Cobra (Figure 18) and the Locust (Figure 32). These always go together. Complete this trio with the Bow (Figure 33) which combines the Cobra and the Locust and follows on. Do the three spinal twists, Marichyasana (Figures 27, 28, 29), and end with Shirshasana, the Headstand (Figure 14).

5. Relax in Shavasana. You are now on your own. Yoga is fun as well as good for you.

8.

WHAT YOU ALWAYS WANTED TO KNOW ABOUT YOGA BUT WERE AFRAID TO ASK

1.   Is yoga some kind of religion?
In India yoga is accepted as one of the *Shat Darshanas* or Six
Revealed Views of Life. It is not in itself a religion but
rather 'the unifying principle behind all religions and
philosophies'. There are today Christian, Jewish, Muslim,
Hindu and Zorastrian Yogis scattered all over the world.

2.   If Hatha Yoga is physical yoga, what is Raja Yoga?
Raja Yoga includes Hatha Yoga. The ancient Rishis
believed that a person's body should be fit and healthy
and under his control before he was able to aspire to
higher things. Raja or Ashtanga Yoga consists of eight
well defined steps. The first four are Bahirang (external)
and consist of Yamas, Niyama, Asanas and Pranayama.
These four constitute Hatha Yoga. The remaining four are
Pratyahara, Dharana, Dhayana and Samadhi, the internal
or Antarang part of RajaYoga. They might be divided like
this:

1.   Yama — Restraints
2.   Niyama — Discipline
3.   Asanas — Postures
4.   Pranayama — Breath control and control of vital
     forces
5.   Pratyahara — Self withdrawal
6.   Dharana — Concentration on one point
7.   Dhayana — Meditation
8.   Samadhi — Enlightenment — the Super-
     conscious state.

3.   Can I practise yoga from a book?
Yes, to a certain point you can. Simple breathing techniques, asanas, and relaxation techniques, combined with
diet, can all be learnt from a book. When you come to
more intricate, higher phases of yoga, you need to learn

from a Guru or teacher, since these cannot be taught by the printed word, picture or diagram. But even if you are learning under a teacher there is great need to take notes, draw small diagrams and generally try and recollect all that has been taught. From this point of view, a book is better. You can keep going back to what you have perhaps not understood perfectly the first time, and you can see the *perfect posture* and try to imitate it. Sometimes you may not realize that you are doing the posture incorrectly. I always recommend that once a week, you get a friend to watch you go through the yoga routine, comparing each posture carefully with the one in the book.

4. Is it necessary to be a vegetarian to practise yoga?
No, not strictly necessary, and many yoga teachers allow their students to eat flesh foods, once or twice a week. But one of the destructive habits in affluent countries is to concentrate almost entirely on meat, fish and poultry — What Dubos calls 'malnutrition of the affluent'. Colonic cancer, heart disease, obesity, diabetes and atherosclerosis are the diseases most prevalent today in developed societies. Yoga also believes in *ahimsa* — non violence, and anyone who practises the higher disciplines of yoga will almost certainly avoid flesh foods which are the dead bodies of once living creatures.

5. Should one give up alcohol, smoking, tea and coffee?
Smoking and yoga simply do not go together and many yoga teachers will absolutely refuse to treat anyone who smokes. His lungs are coated with nicotine and the extended breathing practices will quite certainly harm him rather than improve his condition. Drinking of alcohol every day, or regularly, is similarly a destructive non-habit and should be given up. Tea and coffee, both containing caffeine, are unhealthy drinks, but so are chocolate, cokes and many canned and frozen drinks. All food should be fresh, non-additive (tea, coffee, alcohol and cokes are all addictive) and wholesome.

6. Can the yogic breathing method prove dangerous?
Yes it can, which is why some of the practices must be learnt directly under the instruction of a competent teacher. The practice of the suspension of the breath for

varying amounts of time may have disastrous effects on people suffering from nervous disorders, blood pressure problems, heart ailments and other diseases. According to Tantric texts the object of Pranayma is to arouse Kundalini, the divine cosmic force, symbolized as a serpent coiled and lying sleeping at the base of the spine. The seat of Kundalini lies somewhere between the perineum and the navel; when activated by special breathing techniques and postures, the whole region becomes active on the organs and centres, to effect rejuvenation of the body and elevation of the mind. When learning yoga on one's own it is safest and wisest to keep to reasonably simple breathing exercises which in themselves are of enormous benefit. Shallow and fast breathing habits are changed to slow, deep, complete breathing, oxygenating the blood, calming down the nervous system and providing energy and youth for the body. Deep, rhythmic breathing nourishes and cleanses the body and helps to build up resistance against disease. It also calms and soothes the mind and relaxes the nerves. Anyone looking for more than this must go to a guru in an ashram.

7. Will yoga help my sex life?
Undoubtedly. Tremendous vitality is built up by the various practices and specific postures and Bandhas tone up the sexual centres, the glands which control these centres, and the vital energy stored up by pranayma. Uddiyana and Mula–Bandha (described in Chapter IV) are specially important since the sexual centres are toned, rejuvenated and restored. Yogis use this sexual energy for sublimation, believing that to control such a powerful force gives them psychic powers.

8. How soon should I expect results?
It depends on what you are looking for. If you are looking for a more supple body, greater energy, freedom from disease, a calm and tranquil frame of mind and less tension, you should see results within the first ten weeks, which will improve more and more as you continue your practice. Rejuvenation will take a little longer and will need a steady and continuous practice for ever. Yoga, remember, is a way of life, not something you do for three weeks or a year. The modern world is full of tension.

Doctor's clinics are full of people suffering from psycho-somatic diseases: dizzy spells, asthma, migraine, fatigue, 'nerves', premenstrual tension, insomnia, depression, constipation, chronic diarrhoea, skin eruptions and unexplained aches and pains. Simply by following the routine described in this book, you can cure yourself of all these symptoms. The relaxation techniques are powerful ones, acting like the most potent tranquillizers on the system. The main objective of Yoga is *moksha* — a state of eternal freedom from the cycle of rebirths and therefore from misery and sorrow. This however is outside the scope of Hatha Yoga or this book, but stability and quietness of mind and emotions can be achieved, and a wholistic attitude toward living a life in which destructive feelings and emotions are given up for constructive feelings such as love, friendliness, tolerance and compassion.

9. Will yoga help me to lose or gain weight without dieting?
Yes, this is one of the wonderful effects of yoga. There are asanas, pranayamas and kriyas which speed up the metabolism of the body increasing the rate at which cellular constituents are broken down and recycled for new cellular construction. Internal organs are cleansed and gaseous wastes thrown off with deep breathing. The asanas stretch, twist, pull and lumber up the body which becomes lean and strong. Certain asanas stretch the spine while others work on other parts of the body. In fact there is not a single portion of the body that is not affected by a practice of asanas. Obesity, cellulite, droopy flesh and fat that accumulates on the hips, buttocks and belly are all removed by a sensible practice of asanas, pranayama and Bandhas. If one needs to lose weight then one hour of Hatha Yoga asanas should be practised with the correct breathing techniques and attention to detail. No food should be taken and neither should one take a shower for one hour afterwards, so that post metabolic activity remains high. One should engage in some light activity for this one hour, after which food can be eaten, preferably fruit, fruit juices, some form of cereal, nuts and sprouted grains. Yogurt may also be taken but not with preserved fruits or jams or jellies. Herbal teas with a little honey are good.

If you need to gain weight then also you should do forty minutes to one hour of asanas and pranayamas. These relax the body and provide a form of healthful activity. A warm shower should be taken immediately after a hearty breakfast with cereals, honey, dried fruits, milk and vegetable fats, all eaten in generous quantities.

Yoga also advises you to *think* yourself slim or fatter, and healthier. Think of parts of your body that need changing, either slimmed down or developing some muscle and fat. Think them into a proper shape with positive yogic thinking. One of my pupils, after three months of yoga practice seemed to have slimmed down in all the right places and became extremely attractive. She was naturally delighted with all the compliments but also a little baffled. 'Do you know,' she said to me, 'I haven't lost a single pound in weight. It's just that my weight seems to have settled into the right places.'

10.   Can yoga help when medicine fails?

The ashrams in India and the yogic research institutes are full of people who have been given up by medical science and who have regained their lost health through yoga practices. Diet plays a very important part in these cures as well as asanas, pranayamas and relaxation techniques. Asthma, chronic backaches, high or low blood pressure, constipation and colonic diseases, coronary disease, Diabetes Mellitus, impotency, ulcers, prostatic enlargement, psychic complaints, sterility, spinal deformities, varicose veins, spondylitis (cervical) and numerous other diseases are cured by the practice of yoga. Some yogis also claim the spontaneous remission of cancer after a six-month yoga course. I myself came to yoga through pain. The condition is 'irreversible' said the doctors, as they examined my back. 'Learn to live with it.' But how does one learn to live with such excruciating pain that sitting, standing and walking are agony? Every movement was like a knife stabbing through flesh to bones and muscles. Every activity was torture: it seemed better to be dead. A small book on yoga, picked up at an airport, changed my life. I still meet friends after many years who ask solicitiously about my back pain. Sometimes I stare at them in astonishment. It is so long ago that I have almost forgotten. My spine is today, strong, supple, and more flexible than it was twenty years ago. Perhaps the bone condition, under X-rays may be the same, perhaps not. I have no reason to find out since I am totally without pain and can do a hard day's work and more. The integral science of yoga treats the body wholistically, not as though each part of the body were independent of the whole but as an entire organism, interdependent and integrated.

11. Why does yoga lay so much stress on glandular stimulating postures?
The glands of the human body, such as the adrenals, thyroid, pituitary, pineal and thymus are all responsible for essential life processes. They make us feel vibrant, alive, and far more youthful than our age if they are working properly. But so much can go wrong with the glands. The thyroid can become sluggish, especially after the menopause when the ovaries cease functioning. Women complain of poor memory, develop fluid retention, have a low metabolic rate and there is flabbiness, muscle weakness and loss of muscle tone. The pituitary, the master gland of the body, secretes the hormone which regulates all the other glandular systems. If this does not function, abnormal fat deposits are produced below the waist. There is also loss of hair, loss of sexual drive, shrinking of the ovaries and testes and various other unpleasant ailments. The adrenal glands, the thymus and spleen, the pancreas and the liver all have their vital functions. When there is a breakdown, or when they lose their ability to function, all kinds of serious problems are created. Doctors today are treating glandular deficiencies with dessicated glandular substances and the prostate problems with various minerals, oils and amino acid products. For all these problems yoga has a cure. Some postures are powerful glandular stimulators, forcing the endocrine system to function properly and at an optimum level. The Shoulder Stand, the Headstand, the Cobra, the Fish, Baddhakonasana, Paschimottanasana and Viparita Karani kriya are all excellent glandular stimulators which tone up the glands, pressuring them into activity or slowing them down if they are overactive. The Plough Posture and Uddiyana Bandha and Nauli kriya are also excellent for glandular stimulation.

12.   What can I expect if I come to an Indian ashram to learn yoga?

It depends on the ashram. If you join the serious, dedicated ones, who are not catering specially to Western students (such as Ananda Ashram in Pondicherry and Shivananda's ashram in Rishikesh) then you can expect austerity, discipline, a rigorous teaching programme and untold benefits from your three-month or six-month training programme. An ashram is basically meant to be a retreat from the world, and those who join it are expected to conform to the conditions prevalent there, whether they are Indian or foreign students. For instance, in Ananda Ashram, the moment you enter the gates you will be required to wear comfortable Indian clothes, either the North Indian kurta-pyjama, or lungis or saris. For yoga asana classes you may wear leotards, bikinis, shorts or anything comfortable and appropriate. No meat, eggs, fish, or poultry is consumed and you will be expected to accept this diet in its totality. Much fresh fruit (often from trees in the ashram gardens), fresh vegetables, sprouts, honey, brown bread or unleavened chappatties, seeds, nuts and herbal teas are consumed. The evening meal is taken early, before sunset and is very light, consisting of yogurt and fresh fruit. The discipline is strict and the head of the ashram, the guru, is a benign dictator, in the true tradition of the guru-pupil relationship. The day begins early — usually 4.30 or 5am. The yoga programme is intensive, consisting of hour-long classes of instruction in asanas, followed by much pranayama, and then instruction in yoga diet, asanas, kriyas, mudras, pranayama, as well as Yoga Chikitsa (therapy), yoga health and yoga hygiene. Mantra Yoga, meditation and concentration techniques and Laya Yoga (secret) techniques are taught. The student is expected to do one or two hours every day of Kriya Yoga — some form of work in orchards, gardens, kitchen, office or ashram buildings as part of his progress toward spiritual evolution. One month, three-month and six-month courses are offered. Any student found smoking, taking drugs or drinking alcohol is expelled on the spot. It sounds tough? Nevertheless, hundreds and hundreds of foreign students come every year and often return with their families, to learn at the feet of a true Yogi the true tradition handed down through centuries.

13. Why is there so much emphasis on correct diet and on fasting?

Yoga is a way of life — a method of integrating mind, emotions and body to work harmoniously together. In this, diet plays an extremely important part. Longevity, good health, youthful vigour, good digestion and a body that is nutritionally high in all the necessary substances all work together for total health. Every organ and part of the body is affected by the food that you eat. A diet of whole natural foods rich in vitamins and minerals can fortify every part of the body. Low-fat, high-fibre diets, without refined carbohydrates, fried foods, saturated fats, processed foods and foods that have been sprayed or preserved with additives is recommended. The effect that diet can have on eyes, for instance, is demonstrated by an Indian nature-cure doctor in Delhi, who treats his patients first by changing their entire diets drastically. We sent a twelve-year-old girl to him (we were her local guardians in this town) whose eyesight was deteriorating very rapidly. She had myopia and in one year her glasses needed to be changed as she went from -2 to -4. This doctor put her at once on to a special diet. No meat, eggs, fish or poultry were allowed. She was to eat nothing fried and absolutely no saturated fats. She was encouraged to eat fresh green vegetables either steamed or raw in salads, nuts, plenty of fruits, sprouts, yogurt and cottage cheese, wholemeal (wholewheat) bread and some skimmed milk. No sugar was allowed but two tablespoons of honey was permitted. The honey had to be raw and not processed.

In two months the child showed a remarkable improvement; in six months the number had dropped to less that -2. The improvement continued and when she left here, although she was still wearing spectacles, the number was less than -1. There are also numerous advantages to fasting. The body is rested, and the system is able to get rid of poisonous wastes. Many Indians fast once a week as a matter of routine. Mahatma Gandhi used to say if you have fever, fast, if you have digestive problems, fast, if you have a headache, nausea, pain in any part of the body — fast. Whenever the body is suffering from any kind of illness it is wisest to fast instead of giving the patient milk or broth — both good culture media for bacteria.

Yogis use fasting as a method of keeping the body

healthy and the mind clear and alert. Naturpathic consultants feel that those patients who fast when they are ill, recover twice as fast as those who continue to eat. Many patients have rid themselves of arthritis by fasting and an eye specialist claims that after a fast of four to five days a person is often able to read fine print without glasses for the first time in many years. Generally, in affluent countries, everybody eats too much, with the result that the digestive, assimilative and metabolic processes are grossly overworked. Resting the body by fasting is a very rejuvenating process. The body feels light and energized, the skin is clearer, bloating and gas are eliminated and there is a tremendous feeling of well-being. In all yoga ashrams there will be days of fasting and probably a preliminary three or four days of fast before the training is started. You can eat without counting calories for most of the week if you maintain a fast for one day in every seven days. It enables the body to rid itself of its impurities, gives the digestive system a rest and, if combined with a mild enema, can prove to be one of the most beneficial and health-giving procedures you have ever undergone. The thought of fasting usually frightens a person used to three or four meals a day. Part of your yoga training is to learn to differentiate between hunger and appetite. No one over the age of twenty-five should eat more than his normal lean weight multiplied by fifteen. For instance if you weigh 130 lbs then your calorie intake should be 130x15 which is 1950 calories a day. Most charts recommend much higher calorie intakes but this is the diet at which you will stay fit and healthy. See that the calories are not empty calories but packed with nutrition.

14.   What are the other therapeutical procedures of yoga?

All of these therapeutical procedures must be learnt under the guidance of a competent teacher. It is unwise to try them by oneself. In a yoga ashram many of them will be taught as part of the purifying process of the body. Some are resorted to every single day, some only occasionally. A brief list is given below.

JAL NETI
Jal is water and this is a method of cleaning out the nose which is extremely effective in chronic sinusitis, colds, congestion and stuffiness. I myself have taught this to many sufferers from these troubles, with marvellous results. It is done every morning and prevents colds as well as being good for the eyes.
Technique:
A brass cup with a long spout is the traditional equipment. It is filled with luke-warm water with a pinch of salt. The spout is inserted into one nostril, the head tilted sideways and the water allowed to pour out from the other nostril, flowing from one nostril through the nose and out on the other side. The mouth is kept slightly open or there is danger of choking if water is inhaled.

VAMAN DHAUTI
This is a yogic stomach wash.
Technique:
Four or more glasses of warm water with a little salt in it are drunk down rapidly. The fingers are inserted into the mouth and the soft palate and the pharyngeal wall are tickled. This begins a vomiting reflex and the water is expelled and gushes out. The procedure is repeated until the person feels he or she has ejected the last bit of water. This is excellent for any morning when there is a feeling of having over-eaten or when the stomach feels queasy.

KUNJALI
This technique affects the liver, spleen, pancreas, etc., and is excellent for toning.
Technique:
Saline water is drunk in large quantities as in the previous procedure. An Ujjayi breath is taken with glottis closed and mouth open. The descending diaphragm compresses the stomach and the water rushes out from the throat with great force 'like an elephant'. The stomach is cleansed of all impurities and there is a feeling of lightness and well-being.

VĀRISĀRA OR ŚANKHA PRAKSALANA
In this the whole of the alimentary tract is cleaned out with water. Yogis believe that often the intestines get clogged

with fecal matter and only washing will clean them out.
Technique:
Three or four pints of lukewarm water to which is added
half an ounce of salt and some lemon juice is drunk down
rapidly. Within an hour or two the water with fecal matter
should have been pushed out through the rectum. A yoga
student can help to expedite the passage of the water by
doing certain postures such as the inverted Viparita
Karani which is held for four to five minutes, or the Spinal
Twist is done as well as the Cobra and the Locust. More
water is drunk and the same procedure followed until
finally the entire alimentary canal has been flushed out
and cleaned and nothing comes out but water. The whole
process takes several hours and must be done under
supervision. The student then relaxes, covered with a
light, warm covering and eats a small meal of rice and
lentils or soft cereal. This purification process is often
undertaken if there is some chronic illness or simply as a
routine cleansing process once every three months or so.

VARI-BASTI
This is something like an enema except that the adept
sucks up water through the rectum by control of the
muscles. Others use a tube.
Technique:
The expert squats in a tub or basin of water and using and
controlling the anal sphincters, sucks water up into the
colon. While doing this he performs the Nauli kriya.
When enough water has been taken in, the abdominal
muscles are manipulated, rolling them from side to side in
the Nauli kriya very fast, for a minute or two. The water is
churned inside from the sigmoid to caecum and back
again, cleaning the whole of the large intestine. Unlike
enemas, Basti not only cleanses the entire colon but adds
to the tone as well.

GANESA KRIYA
This is a technique that can be done without tuition and is
especially recommended for older people where the anal
sphincters become dry and there is a clogging of faeces
and a pouching of relaxed muscles.
Technique:
A turmeric root, a finger stall or the middle finger covered

with gauze is used for this procedure. Whatever is used, it is dipped in castor oil and inserted into the anal opening as far as possible, at least three-fourths of an inch. A thorough massage is given to both the sphincters by turning the finger clockwise and anti-clockwise.

All these therapies are usually done in the early mornings before breakfast. For those who have a tendency to overweight these colonic lavages are especially recommended. They are also excellent for expelling toxins from the body.

INDEX